The Day
I COMMITTED
SUICIDE
Memoirs Of A Survivor's Life

Jay Williams

THE DAY I COMMITTED SUICIDE
Memoirs Of A Survivor's Life

Copyright © 2020

New York, New York

Book Project Management—Start Write Publish Team
Layout Design—Inkcept Studio
Photography/Book Cover Design—Bryan C. Greaves, Jr.

All rights reserved.
No part of this publication may be reproduced, distributed, or transmitted in any form or by any means, including photocopying, recording, or other electronic or mechanical methods, without the prior written permission of the publisher, except in the case of brief quotations embodied in critical reviews and certain other noncommercial uses permitted by copyright law.

ISBN: 978-1-64826-071-1

DEDICATION

This book is dedicated to my grandmother Leola D. Smith who always believed, pushed, and invested in everything I did and was my biggest fan before my children were born.

Sleep in Peace
12/19/36-10/3/2009

ACKNOWLEDGMENTS

There are too many to acknowledge in the story of my life. There are so many people that have been instrumental in the making of who I was, who I am, and who I am becoming. However, I will acknowledge God as being the author and finisher of my faith. He called me before the foundation of this world, and even though my life hasn't always been easy, he placed many people in my life at strategic times to shape the woman I've become today. With that being said, He also allowed all things to work for my good. I will also acknowledge my five amazing children who put up with me and have also survived the last seven years of trauma with me. Lastly, a host of family, friends and colleagues. To those who hurt me or caused me harm, I forgive everyone. They did the best they knew how with the resources they had at the time. For this same reason I forgive myself.

FOREWORD

It is so easy to automatically assume that because you've dedicated yourself to being a child of God, that life is going to always be easy. As a preacher, you don't know how bad I would love to stand in front of hundreds and thousands of people and preach a message that guarantees total happiness and sweatless success simply because one has committed themselves to be a child of God. I would love to preach a message, write books, record podcasts and hold life coaching sessions and tell people that when you give your life to Jesus, life is going to be filled with roses, you'll forever walk on water, and your steps will be ordered on lovers lane. If I share that message, it will be a total lie because I haven't experienced that level of bliss in my own life.

Yet, I live with a high level of peace, prosperity, and joy. For some reason, there's an assumption that having a good life means that life is going to be pain-free. That, too, is a lie. I've learned that the peace of God is indeed essential for a life filled completely with joy, but it's necessary not after a storm, but while you're in the middle of a storm. Author Janelka "Jay" Williams is an expert on surviving storms, and assisting people during their most challenging times as well. It's so unfortunate how most people are eager to give up on others when they see them go through a storm. Jay is the type of woman that knows how to shine when things are well, but it's incredible to see after all that she's been through, she still continues to shine.

Moreover, she's shining even brighter today than before. Furthermore, Jay's mental strength has been the key to opening new and more magnificent doors in her life. She has many connections, she's incredibly creative, an excellent communicator, and she's stable in her consciousness. With all of those extraordinary gifts that she possesses combined, the reason why she is still standing, still moving forward, even making a significant impact and shifting lives, is because of her courage. Her life is a perfect example of Romans 8:28, which tells us that all things work together for our good. Her life is proof that you can always "flip the script" and possess complete victory. Actually, the concepts of strength and success have everything to do with how you handle pain while it's present. From heart to heart, and soul to soul, we all have our own individual battles. We have all been faced with unique situations that are sometimes expected, because of our own wrongdoings and the predicted consequence comes at levels higher than what we thought we could prepare for. Then you have the difficulties of life that come unexpectedly, not because of any wrongdoing of our own, but we've been blindsided by the unexpected changes in the people around us in whom we trust.

Many would say there's nothing you can do about that; however, I would say there is something we can do about it, and it's called perseverance. The thought that we are helpless is what sends most of us into a frenzy of panic. Including the proverbial, "I'm losing my mind! "To say that we've never had moments where we've experienced this level of fear or frustration, just because we consider ourselves children of God would be false testimony. I learned even after all that I had gone through, divorce, loss of the baby, financial turmoil, and of course, the discovery of fake friendships, I realize that Jesus had already told us that we would face these unpleasant circumstances. In John 16:33, Jesus says, "I have told you this so that you will have peace by being united to me. The world will make you suffer. But be brave! I have defeated the world!" In other words, it's a guarantee that you're going to have trials and tribulations in life.

Every day is not going to be sunshine. But as believers, we live every day with the confidence that only God can give. We know that all things are working for our good. Every time my wife and I are faced with a battle of any sort, we never lose it! It's just not a part of our lifestyle. We recognize that trouble is a part of our growth. It's all a part of the process. As you read this book, know that the testimony of Jay Williams is real, authentic, and proof that you, too, can be victorious in the middle of a storm.

Marcus Gill
Author, Motivational Speaker
CEO of Marcus Gill International
Myrtle Beach, South Carolina

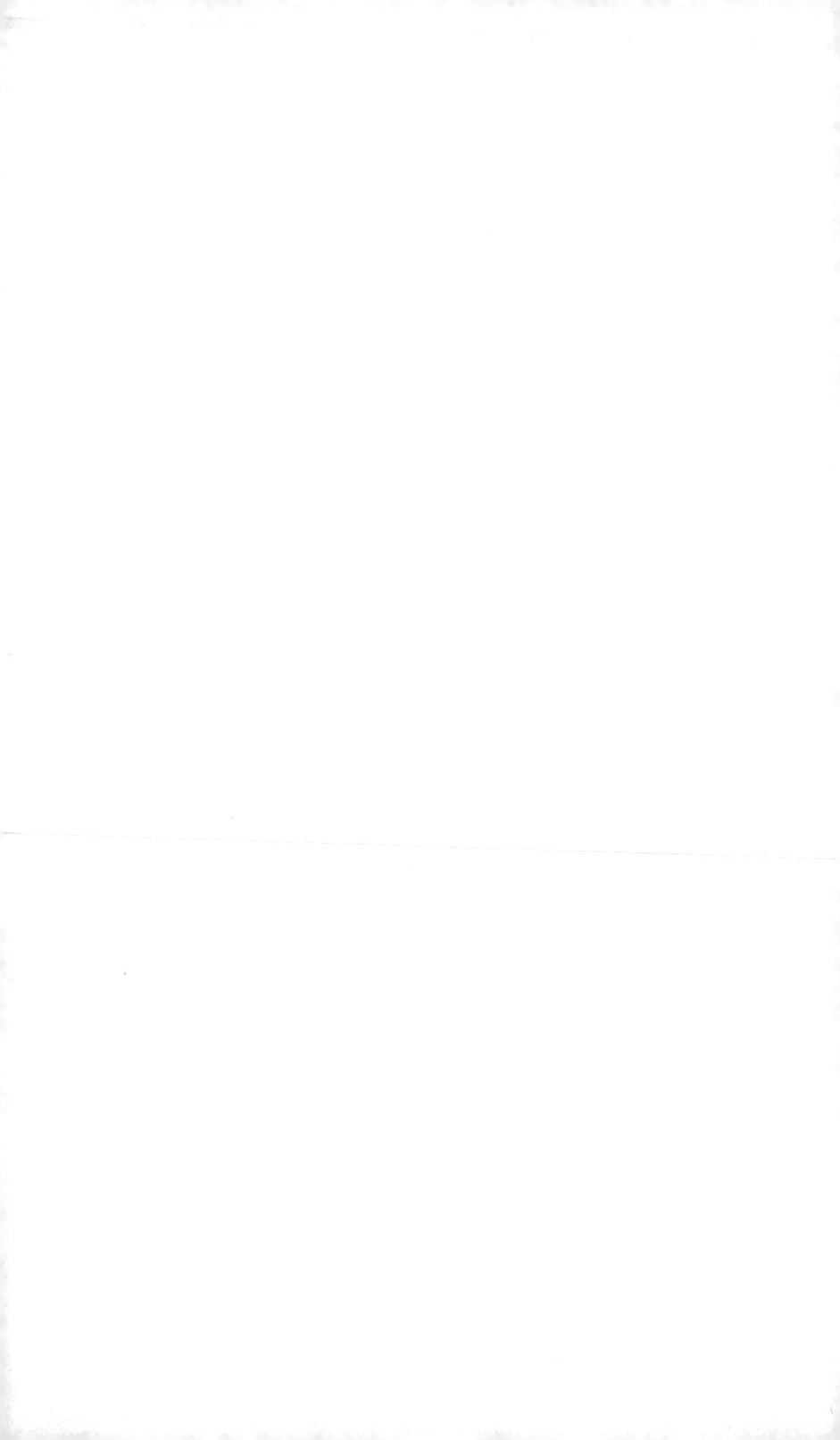

TABLE OF CONTENTS

Dedication 3
Acknowledgments 5
Foreword 7
Chapter 1   *The Turning Point* 13
Chapter 2   *My Childhood: Confidence Created* 23
Chapter 3   *Teenage Years: Confidence Questioned* 35
Chapter 4   *Salvation* 51
Chapter 5   *First Marriage: Confidence Broken* 65
Chapter 6   *Second Marriage: Rebuilding Confidence* 81
Chapter 7   *Pastoring* 97
Chapter 8   *I Knew Something was Wrong: Mental Illness Revealed* 119
Chapter 9   *After That Day* 139
Chapter 10 *The Beginning of the End* 157
Chapter 11 *Rebuilding: The Healing Process Begins* 175
Chapter 12 *Freedom/The Healing Process Continues* 193

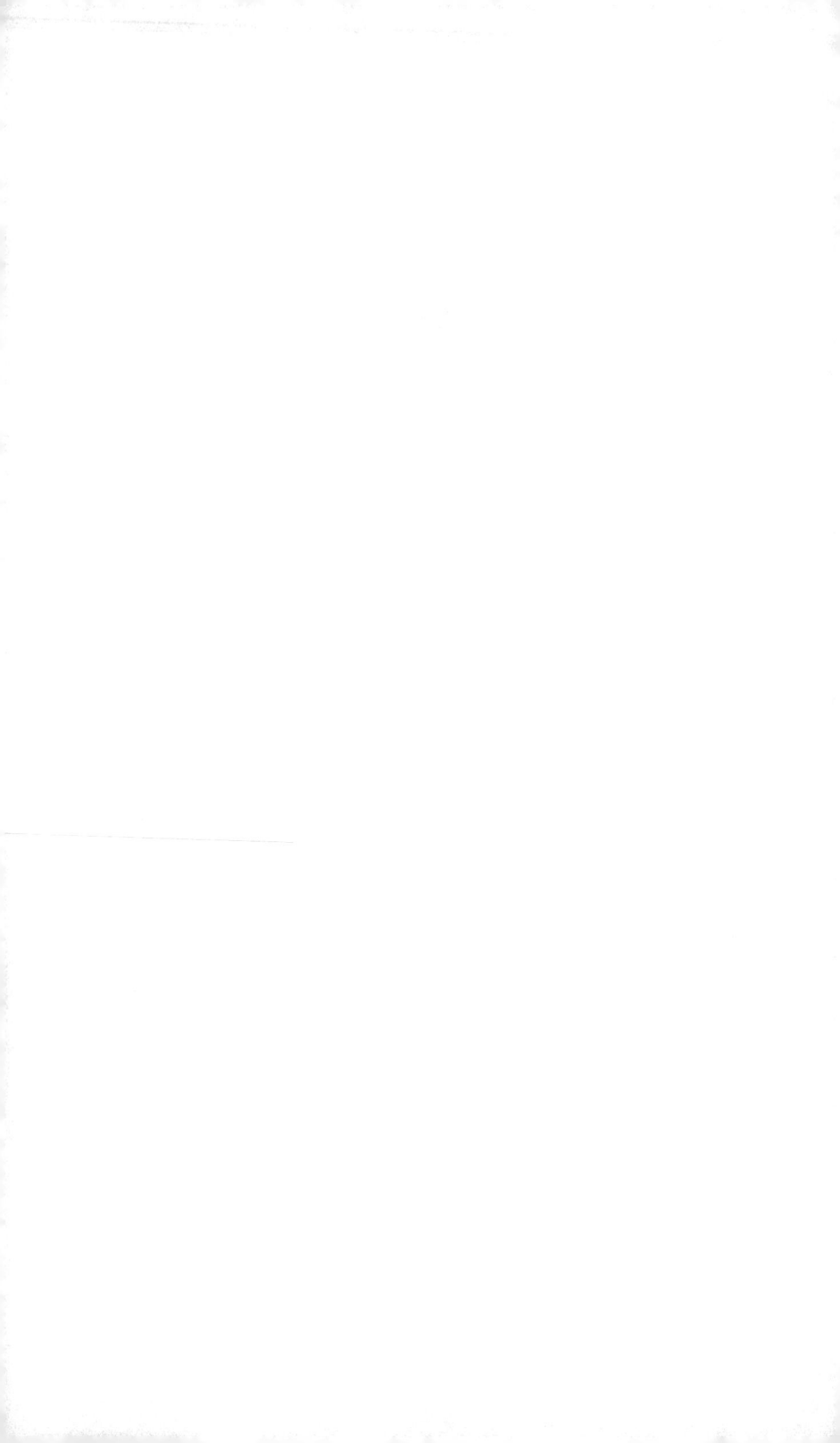

Chapter 1
THE TURNING POINT

September 2, 2017. I will never forget this day. I was running down the stairs, trying to get away from my husband. After three years of badgering me and all of the insanity, I had reached the end of my rope. At this moment of devastation and hopelessness, I decided that it would be better to be with Jesus than to continue living like this.

I felt overwhelmed by the accumulation of stress that I had been enduring for such a long time. I was depressed, and it was growing harder to get out of bed each day to start or complete my daily routine. My best friend was becoming increasingly concerned about me. She knew that something was wrong, but because I was the "Pastor's Wife," I just kept it all to myself. I did not want to expose everything that my husband was putting me through and going through himself.

My best friend noticed that I had been sleeping a lot. She knew me to be a driven and passionate person. But lately, I was losing interest in pursuing any of my dreams anymore. What's worse is that I had no strength or energy to do any of

The Day I Committed Suicide

my caretaking responsibilities for my children and definitely not my wifely jobs since there was nothing that I could do right according to him. I was being made to feel like my "failure to support" him was a detriment to my own dreams and future. Like many women, especially in ministry, the mistake I made was intertwining all of my dreams with my husband's. I was being told by him every day for years that he had given me the world, and I had given nothing back in this marriage.

In an instant, my world seemed to be crashing down on me. I would walk away from him when I didn't feel like fighting or couldn't take anymore. I didn't want to show hurt or pain because he would either mock it or minimize it, and/or use it against me later. However, walking away didn't seem to work anymore--his impulsive need to badger me had become a routine of following me when I walked away to tell me that I'm horrible, nothing and nobody.

All of a sudden, I remembered that I had a full bottle of Adderall and a bottle of medicine leftover from surgery. I decided that today was the day that I would make all the pain stop. I'm not sure how many pills I took, but I just remember taking them all.

My husband watched me take them, all the while, he was still fussing and yelling at me, telling me that I wasn't there for him. When he realized what I had done, he said, "I'm not dealing with this. He went upstairs, closed the door, and never came back out. As I sat down and began processing my exit from life, I started trying to compose a letter. I don't remember the exact words. But I started the note by explaining that "I really tried everything. I mean, I really tried to help, and I really tried to do my best." Then I just stopped. I started imagining my kids coming home from school and me not being there. At that moment, I was terrified of what I had done. So, I stopped writing because and I wanted to call my best friend since I knew that the last month that we were talking, and she was aware of my depression. She knew that I was suffering, even though I had not been ready to open up about it. I realized that she might be able to help. I sent her a text that read something like, "I'm so sorry I did something that I can't take back."

I think she knew immediately from those words that something was wrong, and she called me instantly. My friend was repeatedly asking me, "What happened?" "What did you do?" "What's wrong?"

I was so torn. I wanted to tell her to see if she could help me, but at the same time, I was embarrassed and ashamed to let her know what I had done. Seriously, I'm a Pastor and a counselor; I'm the one that is supposed to help people feel better about themselves and want to live! As a pastor, I preach, teach, and had sessions with women, men, and children to help them develop into becoming their best selves and to never give up. I couldn't find the words to tell her, so all I could manage to get out was, "I just couldn't do it anymore, and I want to tell you I love you." Next, I texted my mom and said, I love you, and I texted my dad and told him that I loved him too.

I will never know for sure (because the shame and uncomfortable topic has never come up again with my children, and I have no contact with my now ex-husband). Still, I believe my husband knew this wouldn't end well, so he reached out to one of my older sons because he appeared out of nowhere, all of a sudden!

And as soon as he got there, he repeatedly began to ask me questions too. "Mom, what did you do? Mom, what did you do?" I couldn't stand to tell him the truth. I was just too embarrassed.

I just whispered, "I didn't do anything." Now, this is one of my older sons. I mean, he was 19 at this point, so he knew something was wrong, but I did not want to tell him what I had just done. Again, a little louder, I spoke up and said, "I didn't do anything." But all I know is that I am shaking inside, I was so scared, but I just couldn't bring myself to tell him that I had taken all of these pills.

Now, my senses are returning to me, and I started feeling like I was crazy to have taken the pills. Everything is crashing in on me, and I begin to cry, thinking about my babies. My younger daughter was in the first grade, and my younger son was in fifth grade. While my brain was exploding, thinking about my kids coming home and being stuck with their father, the man who was causing me pain, I begin to break down. The doorbell rang, and I was crying uncontrollably at this point. The police are there, and they start asking me the same questions, "What's going on? What did I take? How many did I take? How long ago?" The shame that engulfed me had me paralyzed with silence and fear. I was unable to speak. I just remember feeling an overwhelming and profound sense of humiliation and disgrace.

Next thing I know, they are putting me in an ambulance, and at this point, I was totally out of it. My blood pressure was at stroke levels. Later on, I saw a few more of my friends at the hospital. I believe that they were called by my best friend. All I remember is that they looked so hurt. My best friend told me later that I was talking a thousand miles an hour, non-stop. That's what happens when you take something like Adderall.(It's a stimulant like cocaine.)My heart was racing, my pressure was high, and my mind was racing with a million thoughts. You could visibly see the pain on their faces. I still wasn't done facing the people hurt by my actions. I didn't even remember that my daughter was coming home from college that weekend, and she just started crying when she saw me. I have never felt more mortified than I did when I saw my oldest daughter, for whom I've always wanted to set an example of being a strong black woman.

You may ask, "Jay, what in the world brought your world crashing in on you like this?"

Well, I am going to tell you in hopes that it may free someone else. I am sharing these events if, for nothing else, to help others who I believe have had the same experience or will in the future. If I can prevent one person from allowing another person's actions to drive them insane, that is what I want to do!

That Day and 1094 Days Prior

The day that this incident occurred, my husband literally started following me around the house just to tell me how horrible of a wife that I was. He berated and badgered me, continually saying that I didn't support him. For the life of me, I could not understand what I was supposed to be "supporting."

Our lives had slowly spiraled out of control. For two years, my husband was convinced that we were being hacked. For three years, he had started diagnosing himself with a new disease or ailment every week. By the day of this event, he was convinced that he had worms in bizarre parts of his body, and he would become extremely angry with me because when he asked me to look at it, I could not see it.

I had already moved downstairs because I could no longer take him staying up all night. His obsessions went from weight loss to computers being hacked, to being sick, dying, to me being an awful person, to worms in his body. Meanwhile, the whole time this is happening, he's also telling me that I'm the worst wife and mother in the world. For years now, every day, it was another insane obsession or conversation centered on the idea that I was not supporting him. One of the signs that someone is paranoid is they continuously repeat the same words or phrases even when it doesn't make sense in the conversation. It was so off, but because he was well-read and smart, it would sound like it made sense, often driving me crazy. He would often build evidence off of truth and lies to build his case, which made it even more convincing. So much so, you could actually know the truth and have witnessed the truth and still believe his lies.

It didn't happen overnight, but gradually I begin to feel really low in spirit. I would go to church and smile, keep the front and try to hold things down at first. I didn't know I was fighting depression like I mentioned earlier. But, I was blind to it myself. Like many busy moms and ministry wives, I just told myself I was tired. However, this was a "tiredness" that I simply could not shake off. I begin to lose my zest for life and my zeal for ministry, which was just not like me.

When it got horrible, I tried to tell him, my words exactly, "I'm not good." I said it more than once but never did he ever address it. None of my feelings, sicknesses, or exhaustion ever really mattered, and this was before, the manic behaviors. I was always expected to be superwoman or supermom. Cook, clean, take care of him, his clothes, his laundry, the 3600 square ft house, 5 kids, their laundry, their schoolwork, back and forth to the school, make sure every looks good, including myself, help in every aspect of ministry, (because I wasn't the sit on the side and look pretty kind of first lady).

As a matter of fact, it's funny because I left our previous church to start the church with him. When we started our church, I was the usher, greeter, praise and worship leader, and the trustee. Anything that needed to be done, I did it with my whole heart. I built that ministry with him side by side. I made every manual that runs that church, sang for every single service for the last 12 years, and ran several departments. I helped him with his job, but he was unwilling to help with my job, which was the house and kids.

When I married him, I had one daughter, but after a couple years, he decided his boys were moving in with us, and I raised them since they were 8 and 9 years old with very little help from him who threw money at everything that he did not want to help with. I raised them as if they were my own birth children. Then he said he wanted another one so that we can have one together.

So, I gave birth to my son and couldn't work having four children and living 90 miles from my job. Then he wanted a daughter, so at age 33, while pursuing my master's degree, I dropped my educational pursuit and gave him one. So once again, I put away my dreams of doing music and singing, and completing my master's degree, which I was doing at the time, and had a daughter.

Part of the challenge is that, like many young church visionaries, he was battling with his own feelings of insecurity and doubt. He was told that he was not a pastor but an evangelist and that the church wouldn't last for more than a year. He had to fight through the negative words that were spoken over his life, and he promised not to run the church as he had seen with manipulation, keeping people out all week with little family time in an authoritarian leadership style.

In the beginning, everything was great. We were warrior pastors together, momentum was being built as the church was doing phenomenal in its infant stages. We were doubling membership weekly. Folks were being so blessed they would bring 2 or more people back with them every week. I, along with the awesome music department that I led, carried the first half of service, and he preached the second half powerfully. We were often told that we were a powerful duo. But then it became all about him, and what he does, and what everyone else is not doing.

When I think back to running down the stairs. I was so ready to leave. And my despair really was clouding my mind in leaving the house versus leaving the Earth altogether. I just remember wanting, needing desperately to get away from this man who had made me feel like I was the worst person in the world. Meanwhile, I'm trying to explain to him that his ideations were getting the best of him and that he needs to get help. Even with my psychology degree, my husband had me feeling like I was the crazy one because I can't see the worms and eggs invading our home and his body.

In all actuality, I knew he was not well, but in the back of my head, I didn't want to believe that this man was losing his mind. One time, he expressed that he is 99.99% always right and because his "prophecies" seem to never hit the ground, he believed that. When he said it, I felt afraid for him. I told him you better be careful because you are acting as if you sit at the right hand of the Father. It's crazy, but before he began showing signs of mental illness, he arrogantly believed that he was always right and that everyone else around him was stupid. The fact that he was convinced that there are worms in his nails, nose, feet, and his head has to be correct.

I started to look back to the time he became a legit "health nut." There were some manic behaviors taking place at the time that I didn't realize. At first, I believed the weight loss obsession was because he wanted to be healthy. Before that, I thought the beginning of it was when something was going on with the computers. Still, eventually, I questioned, "How is it that for 2 years you're stuck in your office for hours and days at times, spending hundreds of dollars fighting hackers that never really stole anything?" The paranoia grew worse, and then it was worms. He earnestly believed that the worms were everywhere, and when the doctor's testing would come back negative, he was distraught and said the doctors didn't know what they were talking about.

That's just a snippet of what the last 3 years of my life looked like before I decided I could not take anymore. The later chapters of this book will have details that will bring awareness to mental illness and abuse. My culture as an African American woman and a Christian lends itself to me not sharing this story, out of embarrassment and being taboo, as we frequently fail to tell people the things that we go through. However, if we would just make these subjects normal and strive to bring awareness, people would reach out for help and recognize the signs before it's too late. I'm pushing past my embarrassment and fears because, "My passion is that you be well, Spiritually, Physically and Mentally."

Chapter 2

MY CHILDHOOD: CONFIDENCE CREATED

When I look back on my childhood, I wonder how I went from this beloved beautiful chocolate confident child to this vulnerable and fragile being. My dad went to the military, and I think he came back with the baggage of a girl that was writing him and broke off the relationship he had with my mother. They were unable to settle that relationship issue, and I think they broke up and never got back together. When I was born, my mother was 19 and still lived with my grandmother, my aunt, who was 14, and my uncle, who was maybe 17 or 18. Therefore, I was the beloved baby in the house.

My grandmother had a problem with alcohol, and my mother told me when I was older that she didn't always do right by them growing up, but for some reason, I became the precious grandbaby that slept with her, and she spent her time and money on. We bonded because she said I was talking and walking by seven months, and I was so animated, she enjoyed my company.

I was very loved and cherished. My family often tells me stories about my dancing, singing, and knowing every word of every song that came on the radio at one and two years old.

My grandmother adored me and really cultivated my gifts. As a matter of fact, she was a teacher, an artist, who loved everything about the arts. She did all of the performing arts shows at her job, and she put me in her performances at her middle school. Her putting me on the stage at a very early age boosted my confidence. Later, I recall my grandma taking me and getting me an agent that I had to take professional pictures for, and I started going on auditions.

I'll never forget being on an audition with Regina King and Countess Vaughn. Didn't get that gig, though. I often would think back and wonder if I would have stuck with it would I be where those two young ladies are by now. Maybe I would have made it.

Soon after, there was a little rough patch for my grandmother financially, so I stopped going on the auditions, stopped having agents, and my mother began to start moving around. I don't know why we moved so much, but I can say that we moved about 15 times in my childhood from one apartment to the next, at times, and living with other people. I'm guessing a single black mama with only a high school diploma couldn't get a job that paid enough to keep a stable home.

My mother was a really tough cookie growing up. All of the guys in the neighborhood where she grew up were afraid of her. She told me a story about how, when my grandmother moved into the neighborhood in Brooklyn.

At the time, she was one of the few black families to buy a home in that neighborhood.

One day this white girl said something derogatory to my mother, and my mom knocked her out. I guess the white girl went running to her family, and the white boys in the neighborhood came to my mother's neighborhood and jumped my mother. According to my mom, it was about 50 white boys with bats and sticks coming after her. She said all she did was grab one of them and started punching and kicking and trying to destroy his face. In that case, if she got one of them, she was right.

One negative thing about my mother's story is that she was in a lot of bad relationships. As a matter of fact, I remember a time that we were visiting someone in prison that would tell me that I looked like him, and would tell everyone I was his daughter. We went to this place called Greenhaven often and sometimes we would spend weekends there. Now, as an adult, I understand that those were conjugal visits. Later on as an adult, I also realized that was husband number 1. This experience is why I try not to do certain things in front of my children and if I do, I try to explain to them honestly, because when children get older they put the pieces together and realize what was really happening. Don't get me wrong, all parents have their faults, and make their mistakes. The good thing is that both parents and children can learn from them.

After my mom's first marriage, I remember my mother marrying my sister's father. Like my father, he was from Panama. Unfortunately, she married him during the 80s, which was the drug era, specifically the crack/cocaine phase. There is actually a funny story (or maybe not so funny), that I remember. There were some cut up straws on the living room table. I tried to put it up to my nose (probably similar to how I had witnessed my sisters' father and his friend snorting cocaine through straws), and while trying to get it out, it only lodged further up my nose. My mother had to take me to the hospital to get it out. I have told that story numerous times, but now that I realize what the straws were from, it's really a sad story.

My sister was born out of this marriage when I was four years old. The hospital where she was born was one where mostly white people were admitted. So, the day they took me to the window so I could see my sister, there were a bunch of white babies in the clear baby beds. I pointed out the one black baby that was in that room and said, "There goes my sister." Everybody laughed and said, "No, there she goes." I said, "Uh uh, that baby is white; she can't be my sister." Well, to this day, my beautiful sister is lighter than both my mom and her father with light-colored eyes. However, despite her complexion, she looks a lot like my mom.

I remember fighting, arguing, tumbling, and rumbling in that apartment on Ocean Ave. in Flatbush all the time. No one was really going to abuse my mom, but at the same time, there was always a lot of fighting going on, which was scary at times even if she was winning. She said he was a really good guy until he got hooked up on that crap. It just goes to show you how women, even when they are strong, can get caught up in bad situations.

At this point in my life, one of the most traumatic things that I remember happening took place. I think I was about 5 or 6 years old, and when my mother had to work, he babysat me. I don't know why I was home, or maybe I came home after school before my mother got home from work. I can't totally remember; I just recall my sister's dad asking to play with me. My memory recalls being under the covers and him saying, "Let's ride the horse."

I remember him making me straddle him all the time, and I also remember him pulling my underwear down, but I just can't remember if there was penetration. I do; however, remember him rubbing his penis on my vagina. Every day when my mom would come home, I would run in the bathroom, because I always had to urinate after these incidents would occur. One day she confronted me and asked me why I always had to go to the bathroom when she got home. I was afraid to say why so I just said I didn't know. He had told me not to tell, and because of my mother's temper, I wasn't sure if she was going to be mad at me! Well, one day she came home early and caught him, and I ran out.

My mom let me know that she would never let anyone hurt me like that again. She beat his @$$ and put him out. Excuse the typo, it's the best way to describe the whooping he got from my mom. I'm not sure if this was the time, but there was a situation where she cut his hands--almost chopped it entirely off until one of his fingers was hanging off.

I'm telling you my mom was no joke.

I remember one time he came back and snuck in the window and stole all our Christmas presents, most likely to buy his crack. That may not sound like much to some, but I know my mother worked hard to buy Christmas presents. She was not financially stable, and that Christmas, we wound up not having any presents. That is devastating for a child to experience. I can actually still feel the pain that I felt then right now while writing this book.

We moved several times after that. There was a time we moved in with my mom's first husband's mother, an old Haitian lady who looked Indian. I can remember his mother lighting candles and having friends over, with some really weird smells. I now realize that she was doing voodoo. She used to call me skinny and beat me with a skinny belt because I was a picky eater and because me and her granddaughter would get into stuff. Her granddaughter, who I called my cousin, lived with her, and we grew very close. We had fun but I didn't always like getting into trouble. She also used to talk about my light-skinned sister and her pretty eyes. She called her "Grimel." I think that was the beginning of me feeling insecure about being dark-skinned. Because everyone would talk about how beautiful my light-skinned sister was and her pretty green, blue, hazel eyes (her eyes turned according to her mood).

While living there, I would take a private van to my school in Flatbush. During that period, I must have been 7 or 8 years old, and I would dream about a clown attacking me. Whenever I had to go downstairs to take the van, I was afraid that a clown was going to jump out of the bushes before I got to the van. It may not mean that much to some, but that experience was traumatizing to me. That period felt like an endlessly long time in my life. While writing out the events of my life, I realize those reoccurring dreams could possibly be due to the trauma of being molested and seeing all the fighting and abuse that my mother had to endure.

In the African American culture, we don't talk about these things, and so they are never dealt with. We are left to cope with trauma, silently not realizing that it affects our entire life as we move forward. What's crazy is, to this day, I haven't mentioned it again to my mom. I was told not to talk about what happened to anyone. I was told, "what goes on in this house stays in this house." It took me becoming an adult to address it. I would watch talk shows and movies about other cultures who experienced molestation and how they were such a wreck. I would say things like, "Black people go through stuff all the time, and they turn out fine." But as I looked further into my life story, I realize that abuse and the trauma that I've experienced have affected me greatly in a negative way. This may possibly become a discussion once my mother reads this book. And it is a discussion that is necessary.

One time we even moved all the way to Mount Vernon with my sister's father's family. No matter where we moved, my mother tried to keep us in the same schools in Flatbush. The train ride back and forth to Brooklyn was a lot, but also adventurous (if anybody knows about New York City Transit, you know what I'm talking about). I liked it there because it was a big house and I learned a lot about Panamanian culture even if it wasn't my dad's family. Their teenage daughter loved good music, and she knew Heavy D., an up and coming rapper at the time, which we now know to be iconic.

I'll never forget, though, one day my sisters' father came to visit while we were there. I looked at him in disgust. At this point, I think I was a preteen and figured I could actually fight him. I remember deciding to stay away from him at that point.

That was a really traumatic time for me. But that wasn't the last of my mother's husbands. I know that after that marriage she married another guy who was younger than her. His mother was mean and hated my mother. She didn't want him marrying someone with 2 kids. My mom said he was such a momma's boy.

He just seemed so goofy and childish to me because, at this point, I was a teenager. He was so corny to me, and I had an attitude with him all the time. I would backtalk him; therefore, we didn't get along very well. One time I pushed past him with an attitude, and he pushed me over the couch in defense. I will say that it wasn't hard; he wasn't trying to hurt me, but I'm sure he was just annoyed and fed up with me by then. This was crazy of me because he was like 6'4" tall and weighed almost 300 pounds. I guess at this age I wasn't trying to adjust to a new father. Those changes were a lot. It's bad enough I didn't get to see my own biological father who she never married. The first husband we had to visit in jail, then the second husband is on crack /cocaine and molesting me. Now I have to deal with this young guy, who I found to be very petty and childish. I think as women who are single parents, we must take into consideration that when we move from relationship to relationship, you are not the only one that is enduring the effects of these bad relationships. Your children are too.

When I was 14 years old, we had moved from Flatbush to Brownsville, and there was already a lot of adjusting for me. Then my little brother was born, and I had a lot of responsibility in helping with him. Additionally, on top of the fact that I had to take 4 trains with my little sister to get back to the school, I used to attend. Since my mom liked the schools in Flatbush and didn't want to move our schools every time we moved, no matter where we lived, we still attended the same schools in Flatbush.

This was a good look on my mother's part because although I could not make and keep connections where we lived, there was some stability in staying in the same school district and keeping my friends in school. Plus, I don't think I could have survived the Brownsville/East New York Public Schools. Brownsville and East New York were worse than "Bedstuy do or die" back in the '80s. Shootings and stabbings were always being reported in those schools. The schools I attended would have fought every day, but we still only used our hands in junior high school.

One day while going to school, I lost my sister on the train. That was one of the scariest days of my life because I knew how protective my mother was. Fortunately, my sister knew the routine, and when we got separated in the crowd, she just took the train and kept on going to the school. That was a very traumatic day for me, because I thought I had lost my sister and that my mom was going to kill me. After calling the cops and the school we figured it out. My friend at the time who lived way out in Brownsville/ East New York with me and traveled to go to our school in Flatbush like me, was then commissioned to help me hold on to my sister from that time forward. It's crazy because after losing touch after middle school, I found out that she was my second husband's cousin! I learned this while we were at his father's birthday party, trying to reconnect with that side of his family.

So, my childhood was a bit of a roller coaster. I found out that my sister's dad had gone back to Panama and that they helped him get clean, but he died a few years later because his organs couldn't survive the sudden shock of not having drugs. At least that is what we were told. I didn't know how to feel about that. My sister didn't react to her own dad's death because she never really knew him. And as adults, when I told her what her dad had done to me, she was shocked, but I also believe this affected her negatively. My sister and I actually never spoke about the molestation after that, and I think there was an unspoken agreement that we should never talk about it or tell anyone. When I look back, I know that it affected my mother. She became an over-protective parent that would not allow us to do anything. She wouldn't let us go to sleepovers--she wouldn't even let us go outside! I had to figure out my own ways to have fun at home, and when I got old enough, I would just cut school all the time.

Throughout my early years, I remember my grandmother always being around for significant events like birthdays and stuff like that. Whenever our family fell short financially, she always came through for us. I had such an excellent relationship with her. The things that I really wanted that my mom couldn't afford, my grandmother would buy for me. There were times my grandmother said she wasn't going to give me the money for something I wanted and all I had to do was say, "Please Gramma" a few times, and it was done—so much so that my mother would always get annoyed and say that I was her favorite.

I still had the shows and performances that made me happy and confident. I made the lead part for Diana Ross in the Black History Month show in public school amongst other plays. My grandmother continued to cultivate me and put me in shows at her school.

One day I got into a fight with another girl because I made the audition for the talent show at my junior high school. The girl and her cousin followed me home after school and tried to jump me, but I knew if I could just get to my mother, I would be okay. They were both twice my size, and her cousin was 2 grades above me. They were cursing at me all the way home in their intimidating Jamaican accents. I got to my mother, and the same girls who were cursing me all the way up and down the street had a different tune when they saw my mother. When the older cousin realized that that was my mother I ran to, she said, "Oh, you going to beat up a little girl?" My mother said, "First of all, you are bigger than me, and second of all if you are going to be up in my face like a grown-up, I' ma beat you like a grown-up." She probably thought my mom was my sister, like most do because my mom always looked young for her age. This is why growing up, I always felt we'd be okay because my mother was a fighter and not afraid of anybody or anything. As kids, we always see our parents as superheroes, not realizing they are human beings too.

She loved and protected us, but after the baby stage, there wasn't a lot of hugs, kisses, and "I love yous." There was a lot of beatings, cussing out, and struggles. Her overprotection felt like a prison and I assumed she hated me because I got the most beatings and cuss outs I guess because I talked a lot and always had to have the last word. To this day, I don't just take what people say; I ask questions, and I research what people tell me. My sister was quiet, and my brother was the beloved baby son, so they didn't get in as much trouble. We finally planted ourselves in Flatbush when I was 14 in an apartment; my mom still lives there to this day.

No matter what my mom started young, and did the best she could with the resources she had at the time. I know without a shadow of a doubt she, loves, supports and protects her children. Her childhood was shaky, my dad childhood was shaky, who knows what their parents childhood consist of. This is why once we are older we should appreciate and respect our parents no matter what we've been through. We never know why they made the choices they did. My parents are my biggest supporters and protectors today. I could only wait and embrace what my children will say their childhood was like. However, what we all must do is learn from it, either what to do or what not to do.

Chapter 3

TEENAGE YEARS: CONFIDENCE QUESTIONED

As my siblings were born, I remember getting into trouble all the time. Honestly, I had a big mouth and talked back a lot. But I also took the brunt of all trouble because I was the oldest. When I was in the 7th or 8th grade, I had my first boyfriend, and it was tough because the abuse I suffered made my mom super restrictive. I couldn't go anywhere, and I couldn't hang out with my friends. I began to resent her because everybody was having fun after school and on weekends, but I couldn't. So, I started getting really creative to orchestrate my own fun.

This was when I began to cut school all the time, and I started to get into real trouble. I would hang at hooky parties with my friends and my boyfriend at the time. This is where we snuck out of school and went to a friend's house whose parents weren't home and partied. I even got into a fight one time with a girl and got suspended from school. That was something else because I was winning but when the girl got a hold of my long ponytails she started to pull my head down and my best friend jumped in to get her off my hair. She only jumped in to get her hands off my hair and jumped out, but we all were suspended. She had been my bestie since third grade, and to this day, when we catch up, it's like we never lose touch.

Back when I was in middle school, you could tell who was in the smart class because if you were in sixth grade, your classes were numbered 6:1 through 6:14. With the numbering system, 6:1 was the SP (smart class), and 6:13 and 14 were the special education classes. As an educator, I look back and see that this was a horrible system and one of the reasons why children in special education were made fun of, killing their self-esteem, most likely scarring them for life. In sixth grade, I was in 6:1. The next year, in the seventh grade, I was in 7:4. After cutting school at the end of that school year, when I was in 8th grade, I wound up in 8:10 or 11. I can't remember exactly, I just remember it being a disgrace. My mother used to say, "I know your dumb @$$ is smart, you're just not going to school." That was the beginning of me being on punishment throughout the rest of my school years. SMH.

Now going into high school, all of my friends were going to Erasmus, which was near my middle school. But my mom used my grandmother's address and put me in South Shore High School in Canarsie, which was miles away from my neighborhood. She wanted me to get away from what she thought were bad influences. I didn't know anyone, but of course, I met some friends that were freshmen like me. I never really had a tough time making friends. I'm very outgoing, warm, friendly, love to have fun and laugh, and the fact that I was talented always drew people to me.

Nonetheless, I think that was the time around when I started feeling self-conscious about my looks because both of my girlfriends were light-skinned. If you know anything about the 80s and 90s in black culture, having light skin was the in thing at the time. When boys would try to talk to my light-skinned friends, first, I reverted back to my feelings when my sister was born with fair skin and green eyes, and whenever we went anywhere, there were always comments about "that pretty little yellow baby." So, I had probably blocked it out of my mind until high school where a bunch of my girlfriends always got all of the attention, because not only did they have light skin, but they were shapely with boobs, butts, and hips. I had none of that; I was just a skinny little black thang.

But that was not my only issue. Being too talkative kept me in trouble. This had my mom fussing at me all the time. If I wasn't talking, I was singing around the house. My uncle tried to pay me to be quiet when I was little, and I couldn't do it. My mom liked the way I sang, but she said I was always singing and it was loud; and in a small apartment, I guess it could get annoying. So, I was always being told to shut up. The good thing was that my mom loved music, especially R&B. So cooking, cleaning, and getting ready for events were always done with the latest music playing. I didn't get told to shut up then because the music was playing louder than me. I even formed singing groups with my sister and cousin or my high school best friend who would hang at my house all the time, where of course, I sang lead.

One of my fondest childhood memories was taking that walk to Flatbush Avenue on the corner of Cortelyou Road to the record store to buy the latest music releases. I also grew up partying. My mom had a big party with a D.J. every year for her birthday. This why I love good music, dancing, and having a good time. You can never take away from me. My mom had drinks at the party, but she never drank, smoked, or did drugs. I truly respected that and decided to follow in her footsteps. And we partied harder than those who were under the influence.

My high school best friends and I joined the high school gospel choir where I got to lead a couple songs. This experience brought me back to my grandma, taking me to church. She said I cried to lead the adult choir when I was just 3 years old. I don't know why I stopped going to church with my grandmother; therefore, I'm not one of those preachers or churchgoers who can proudly say that I grew up in the church.

I used to sing up and down the hallways in high school. I would even sing in the lunchroom for my friends. I had all Whitney Houston and Mary J. Blige songs down pat. My friends would say, Wow, you sound just like them!" I would also try to tackle some Mariah songs. One time a friend of mine asked me to come to the studio because he was trying to start his rap career, so I went, wrote, and sung the hook. I don't know whatever happened to that, but that would be the first of many studio visits that never went anywhere for me.

Now even though I know my mother loved us, she's always been a little sharp with her tongue. She'd call us names; I mean, my mother had a very derogatory vocabulary. Actually, my whole family does. She always told me if my head wasn't attached to me, I'd lose it because I was forgetful and would sometimes lose things. There were things that I didn't know, but I don't think she realized it was because it wasn't taught. I found myself in my adult life getting upset with my kids about stuff that I never taught them. How can I expect them to know something that I didn't train them to do? As a result of growing up with a very confrontational mom, I have shied away from people who were too rough with their mouth or people who I felt would try to make me feel like I was stupid.

My mom used to say things like, "Your looks are not going to get you everywhere." At family events, I was told I was a "pretty chocolate girl." But my mom would always tell me that my dad "thought his looks were gonna get him everywhere, but he ain't got a pot to piss in or a window to throw it out of" (if you grew up with a black mama you might have heard this before). "You got to finish school," she would say, "You got to have more and do more than be pretty." This was good advice; however, it caused conflict with me not having my father in my life. Then to be accused of being just like him was daunting. Psychologically, when there is a parent absent from your life, there is a void, and you suffer from identity issues. Essentially there are parts of you that you don't understand because there is a part of you missing.

I saw my dad once in a while at events because everyone that grew up in that Brooklyn neighborhood where my mom grew up stayed friends. They support and celebrate each other to this day. It's a beautiful bond, and they are truly "framily" (friends that became family). Every time I transitioned from neighborhoods, schools, and life, I lost contact with the people I had grown close to. It actually explains why this pattern has continued to the present day. My dad also grew up in that neighborhood, so I was able to see him at times during family events. I call them the Troy Avenue Crew.

When I did see my dad, I remember being very happy. He was handsome, and I looked just like him. He was charismatic and very funny. He was so proud to say he was my dad. He would tell everyone, "Look at my daughter, she gorgeous just like her dad." Yeah, he was conceited and just knew he was God's gift to women.

Nonetheless, it was confidence-building for me, because all girls need to hear from the first man in their life that they are beautiful. He would boast about my talent to everyone. He was definitely a proud dad. I do remember him saying he came to get me to see his mom once when I was around 2 or 3 years old, which was a struggle because when I was very young, my mom didn't really let anyone take me anywhere. I have a scar from a gash on my right eye for trying to dance for them and falling on a glass table. He said the fear he had to go back and let my mother know what happened was terrifying for him. His mom was born in Panama to Jamaican and Grenadian parents. My dad said when my grandmother got pregnant by a Navy guy, she didn't tell him. So, he got back on the ship and sailed home, never to find out he had a son. Therefore, my dad never met his father. My grandmother emigrated to America when my father was only five years old. My grandmother later became a Jehovah's Witness and married a really mean Basian man, who my dad, in my older age, has told me the heartbreaking stories of his abuse at the hands of this man. I didn't get to know her really well; therefore, I didn't know all of this growing up.

On the other hand, I see why my mother was annoyed with him. He would make her laugh when he saw her too, but she was a struggling single mother with three children from three different dead-beat fathers. Her life was far from easy. There was a lot of dysfunction. It's not until you get older that you realize how much dysfunction you had going on in earlier parts of your life. It's not until you're educated, and you are aware, or you see a more functional family that you realize yours was a mess. And don't start watching these makeshift TV shows like the Cosby' s—those shows will make you think your life was the absolute worst compared to them. Then there's the other stage of life when you realize everybody has some form of dysfunction growing up. Everybody grew up differently and has a different perspective on how life should be. That's where I'm at now— I'm grateful for all of my experiences; it shaped who I am today. And I don't think I turned out that bad.

In the 10th grade, I was fully adjusted to South Shore High School, and there was this Trinidadian guy who was hanging out in the hallway or the lunchroom (I can't remember which one). He would always call me sexy, and make comments about my beautiful smile, sexy legs, and pigeon-toes stance. He was persistent even when I was paying him no attention. Like most women, I pretended not to care, but I would actually look forward to passing him by to hear what charming thing he had to say next. Over time, I caved. I could no longer take his amazing compliments, and continue to ignore him. I gave him my number and we started talking on the phone all the time. This was during the time that if someone was on the phone and another person was trying to call in, the phone was busy. Oh, and that was the house phone because cell phones weren't widely accessible then. We're talking 1993. So, if someone told my mother that they called and the phone was busy, I would get into big trouble. And don't let her be expecting a call! She would pick up the other phone and say, "Get off my phone, I'm expecting a call!" This was very embarrassing, but anybody from that time knows that if you were a teenager, you went through the same thing.

So now this Trinidadian boy and I are talking every day, hooking up in the hallways, making out, and getting very close. I was his girl, and he wanted to see me outside of school, but because my mother was really strict about me going out in the evenings and the weekends with friends, I never even bothered to ask if I could go on a date. So instead, we would just play hooky from school, and I would go to his house. This was when I lost my virginity. It wasn't like the negative experiences that I heard my other girlfriends talking about, with it hurting and being quick. That experience was amazing, and he made it and made me feel special. He was a few years older than me, so I guess he was experienced and knew what to do. What I'll never forget is that he was playing R. Kelly's, "Sex Me." I fell in love with the artist and the album that day. With him being a few years older than me and very experienced, the whole music choice and experience is a bit taboo. Either way, I still remember it being a great experience that went on for months, but as a teenager, it felt like years.

One day during booster practice, (one of the cheerleading teams consisting of all black girls doing "step" or as we would say keeping the beat--the cheerleaders and twirlers were mostly white) one of the older girls, made mention that the guy I was talking to had a girl that they called his wifey. When I confronted him, he said that he had been over. But as I was doing a little investigation, I saw her in an outfit that totally matched something he wore before. It was dark blue denim, "Guess" jacket and jeans. If they had matching outfits, she must have been wifey. To this day, I don't know if they were still talking to each other, but I did not like the idea of my man having a history before I came to the school with someone considered his wifey. It was scary to me, and I didn't want anything to do with him anymore. So, I cut him off immediately.

He was so upset that he would come up to the school even though he barely went anymore because he was outside selling drugs. But, he would wait outside for me and say, "Janelka, please girl, I miss you." I didn't care. I didn't want anything to do with it. When I look back, I see that it was my fear of rejection and my inability to stay attached when I'm afraid.

Shortly after that ended, I met another really nice Trinidadian guy. We exchanged numbers, and we spent a lot of time on the phone. Next thing you know, we were in the hallways hooking up and making out. The other guy found out and almost got into a fight with my new guy. He was such a savage. He also showed up at my doorstep and at my school bus stop a few times. He was relentless, but I told him I didn't want no parts of him.

My new guy was such a sweetheart. I decided that I would continue our relationship on the phone only. After a while, we would slip out of school for hooky parties here and there. But I wasn't going to make the mistake of giving my body again, not knowing where the relationship was going. I really liked this guy, and people were actually calling us the "in" couple, saying I was his wifey. I liked that status. I'm sad to say that during that year, he got caught selling and got locked up. I remember being really sad, crying at my aunt's house during the holidays, but there was nothing I could do.

We lost track of each other, and never hooked up again after that. I did talk to a couple of guys after that but nothing serious; just phone calls, and hookups at my god-sister's house who lived near my school. I enjoyed flirting and talking to guys, but I was now fearful of hooking up seriously with anyone if it was only going to end in me losing them.

At the end of 11th grade, I used to hang out with a bunch of West Indian girls. I told everybody I was Panamanian, but everybody thought I was Jamaican or Trinidadian. My best friends were Jamaican and Haitian. The truth is I was American raised by an American woman, but for some reason, living in Flatbush, where most West Indians migrated, I quickly picked up on the West Indian culture. Now I know it was in my blood because when my grandmother died, she told me that her father was from Jamaica and her mother was from Grenada. They married and migrated to Panama so that my grandfather could work on the Panama Canal. They then had several children, and of course, my grandmother had my father in Canal Zone, Panama.

I don't know how this beef got started, but all I know is that there was a beef between the West Indian girls from Flatbush and the American Brownsville girls. Girls were getting sliced up here and there. Those Brownsville girls were no joke, and although I had nothing to do with its infant stages of this beef, Brownsville girls were coming after the West Indian girls whether they were in the group that started the beef or not. So, one day my naïve self grabbed some kitchen knives from my house and brought them to school to protect myself.

This was such a dumb thing to do. That year one of our football players was stabbed and killed, and they installed metal detectors in the school and would perform checks randomly. Now, every day prior, I had gone to school and was never selected to go through the metal detectors. But on THIS day that I decide to bring kitchen knives to school, I was asked to go through the metal detectors. As a result of bringing the knives to school, I was suspended and had to attend suspension court on a later date. During that court case, my mother decided that this school was not conducive to my learning experience and put in a petition for me to be put in one of the best schools in Flatbush: Midwood High School. Talk about hurt! I had to leave all my friends and start attending a new school where once again, I would not know anyone. Well, that didn't turn out to be the case because since it was in Flatbush, I did know a few people.

One of my best friends met a guy that lived near my house, and that guy had a friend who showed interest in me. He was another Jamaican, but he was a lot more Americanized.

When I first met him, I thought he was so cute. Unlike my Jamaican friends wearing "Damage" and "Used" name brands with a pair of Wallabee boots, this Americanized Jamaican was wearing a Ralph Lauren sweatshirt with a teddy bear on it with Girbaud jeans and Eastland boots. He was super cute with a shy countenance. I always seemed to attract the shy, yet observant type. They loved my outgoing personality, so they would say.

Now, after lengthy talks on the phone, we decided to hook up at his house just once. I remember bleeding during intercourse. I initially thought my period had come back because it had just ended. Later on, I started to think my hymen broke, because that never happened with my first intimate experiences with my first. After months passed, I realized I hadn't gotten my period. Yes, I was pregnant. After one time with this guy.

I called and told him about the pregnancy, and he seemed pretty scared about it. He also mentioned that we were young, and we probably couldn't handle a baby right now. He was right, but I was the one that was pregnant, and I had to make this decision on my own. I hid it from my mother until I was nearly 4 months pregnant. But let me pause about the pregnancy for a moment, because at the same time, other things were happening.

While I was pregnant with his child, he got shot in the neck by a friend. I'll never forget going to the hospital to see him while being pregnant. I was worried and traumatized, thinking I was going to lose my baby's father before I even had the baby. Although that relationship was short-lived, it's one I'll never forget due to all of the traumatic events that occurred during that relationship. Thankfully, the bullet went in and out his neck, not hitting any major arteries, and he recovered pretty well.

Now one day, I was poking out, and my mom just happened to notice and was like, "Girl, are you pregnant?" Plus, I was eating like crazy, which wasn't really unusual; I was always a skinny fat girl. I was unable to deny it anymore, and she was really pissed, but not ready to beat my behind like usual. She just sat me down and said, "Listen, you can't afford no baby, and I sure can't afford to help you with another mouth to feed in this house. So, what we are gonna have to do is go down to the clinic and get rid of it." I cried and said I didn't want to, and that's when she really got upset; she yelled and let me know that I wouldn't be able to stay there if I had the baby. She went so far as to invite my boyfriend over, and together they were trying to convince me not to have the baby. I don't even know why I wanted to have the baby, I just did. But after days of going back and forth with her, I decided I had no other choice. I wasn't going to get the support from the baby's father nor my family anyway.

When I got to the clinic, I had to do all this paperwork and bloodwork, and I remember being so scared. When they called me in and asked me was this my choice, I let them know it wasn't. After crying hysterically and telling them that I didn't want to do it, they sent me home. As soon as we got to the doors of my house, my mother began to get some bags and started packing for me to leave. The reality hit me: I had no money, no diploma, no job, and no place to go. I told her that we could make another appointment and I would go. Long story shortened, I went back to the clinic at 5 months pregnant. At this point in the pregnancy, it had to be a two-day process. They had to insert sticks inside of me, which was very painful. And when I went back, the procedure was done. I was sad for a very long time after that. I wasn't a Christian at that point in my life, so there was no conviction about abortion, but the loss of my baby that was growing inside of me, was heartbreaking for a very long time. That baby would have been about 25 years old now. Yes, I still keep count.

I met my next boyfriend at Midwood High School. He was one of my best boyfriends. He was a good student and had a job as a barber. And because I had messed up so much in the first 3 years of high school, I had to do a lot of work to graduate, but he made sure I got my schoolwork done and on time. He was a great boyfriend. I was in night school 4 nights a week my entire senior year and had a 0-9 period schedule when most seniors had a 2-4 period schedule. I guess because I was older now, I introduced my boyfriend to my mom, and she let me go out on dates with him. There was a sexual relationship, but it was cool. He gave me all kinds of jewelry, and did I mention he was Panamanian? I loved this because I was getting a taste of my heritage. He was a real Panamanian, and even spoke Spanish. I loved our relationship, and he worked at the barbershop at the corner of my house. So, after school and doing homework, I would hang out at the shop. Passing by all the corner boys hollering to see my man who was working felt like a boss move. He would then get off of work and hang at my house.

I was still cutting school at times to be with him, but not as much as in the past. However, my school let me know that I wouldn't be graduating with my class. This was the year they started the rule that would not allow seniors to walk with your fellow classmates at graduation if you didn't have all of your credits by the actual date of graduation. This really sucked, because then my mother decided I would not be able to join in on the senior festivities. At the same time, my grandmother paid my senior dues and bought my senior ring, but my mother said I could not go to my prom. I thought this was a little unfair because I had really worked hard by going to night school, and I had caught up a lot by only needing two more credits to graduate. This was an incredible feat--I should not have been able to catch up that much because I hardly went to school my entire sophomore and junior years.

My boyfriend bought our tickets to the prom, but she still wouldn't let me go. To this day, I'm hurt about this. You can never get your senior prom back. I went to summer school and got my diploma which reads August 1995. I graduated in the right year, just not the right month. I still think I should have been able to go to my prom. What's cool is my grandmother started the tradition of giving her grandchildren $500 as a graduation gift. I was still able to receive that in August.

Looking back now, I see that my abuse at a younger age, resulted in me engaging in sexual relationships at an early age. I didn't really see anything wrong with it at the time. My back to back relationships were the result of me looking for love and attention from boys. It's clear to me now that the kind of abuse I experienced did have an effect on me even if I didn't acknowledge it. Some form of therapy should have taken place so that I could deal with what happened and gain an understanding of the trauma and its' effects instead of seeking healing in unhealthy ways. With that being said, without this knowledge, the dysfunction continued into adulthood.

Chapter 4

SALVATION

When I was 14 years old, we moved next door to one of my mom's oldest friends. When I say one of her oldest friends, I mean, they had been friends since they were nine years old. She was part of that Troy Avenue Crew that I mentioned earlier. I didn't know it then, but this would be the last stop for a long time. My mom actually still lives in that Flatbush apartment. I remember we started out in the apartment across from her friend on the first floor and then eventually got the bigger apartment beside hers, still on the first floor, but with 2 bedrooms instead of 1 bedroom, the apartment in the front of the building.

After moving there, I ended up seeing my mom's friend's son. I hadn't seen him for a while, maybe since my 10th birthday party with all of my friends going crazy talking about, "Oh my God, he's so cute!" He's always been very tall, dark, and handsome. I was just proud to call him my big cousin. I called him my cousin because for a short time while I was in kindergarten and first grade we were in the same school. He was in the upper grades, so he became like my protector. My time at P.S. 135 didn't last long because while we lived down the block from the school, my mother would bring me to school late every day. Whenever I went into the room, the teacher in my first-grade class would ask, "Why are you so late?" That alone was questionable because if I'm only six years old, I'm obviously not bringing myself to school.

One day the teacher got fed up and decided that she was going to make me stand in a corner for an entire day because I was late for school. A six-year-old standing in a corner for a whole day-just imagine that! Well, I'm sure you already know, Jay's mom doesn't play that! The next day my mom was up there, giving this teacher the business. I will not repeat all the choice words my mother gave that woman that day because I'm trying to keep this book as clean and classy as possible. I remember the woman having so much fear in her eyes. And after talking to her, my mother went to the principal and told her if she messes with my daughter again it's going to be a problem.

After that day, I remember being treated funny by this teacher for the rest of the school year. And then, she put me in a special education class for second grade. My mother was so appalled that she decided to pull me out of that school and put me in a school in Flatbush, where she later got an apartment. I was afraid to start a new school, but I met one of my best friends that I still love to this day; and I had one of the best teachers ever, who put me in my first play in school, where I played Diana Ross. I met one of the most incredible music teachers, who happened to be one of the only black women in the school. I also found out the school PS 139 was later named after that music teacher, the Alexine Fenty School.

I remained in Flatbush schools until 8th grade, no matter where we moved to in New York.

But, getting back to moving next to my mom's friend. Her son would come over and check us out sometimes. He would always ask me to sing, saying, "We need you at my church, singing." I would tell him, "Trust me, you don't want me at your church because if I walk in the doors, the church is going to burn down." Now, I was nervous and hesitant about going to church because I was "that girl" from high school that was living "that life." You know, 'ratchet' is what we would call it today. He kept telling me I need to be in church, and my mom was really on board with it. I kept trying to leave my mom and go live with my aunt. I actually moved in with her, but that didn't really work out because her boyfriend was not cool with it. It was too many women in the house for him. So, I was back with mom for a short while.

After having an abortion, I realized that I needed something more; that I had an inner void. I finally decided to take him up on that offer and go to church. We were telling everyone we were cousins because that's what we had been saying for years. Well, no one was feeling that because they had never met this cousin, and he grew up in that church. He picked me up every Sunday and brought me home. So, I never missed a Sunday, because I was riding in the car with him.

Once I started coming regularly, I started experiencing a little hate from some of the other young ladies there. I guess it was because I got to hang out with the pastor's son. Also, keep in mind that he was tall (6'4" now), dark-skinned, and handsome, so needless to say, a lot of the young ladies in the church were interested in him.

I joined the choir and enjoyed it so much. There used to be little solos given, and I managed to get one. And you know, the jealousy I experienced really kind of shocked me. Honestly, since I was coming from the world, I thought that everybody in the church was going to be kind and loving people. I thought I would be getting away from the craziness of the world, and that when I came to the church, everyone would be genuinely loving.

I couldn't believe how mean and rude some people were in the church. It was not a good feeling. I mean, I remember singing in choir rehearsal and someone turning around and yelling, "You're too loud!"

One of the young ladies told me later that she was a little salty with me because when I first came, they had put me in the gospel rap group as the lead singer, which was actually her role. But she was never told that they were taking off the group. I just came in that day singing the song that she was supposed to be singing and no one said anything to her or me. Months after, we had a conversation about it, and I felt so bad. Fortunately, we were able to overcome that situation and became friends. I would hang out at her house all the time, eating her mom's Jamaican food.

As I matured as a Christian, I realized that everybody in the church is human, flawed, and has issues. The expectancy of the world is that everybody in the church is good, kind, and perfect. But just like I was sitting in the church and a newcomer, someone may have sat next to me and experienced my immaturity as a Christian and could have been hurt and offended. Either way, it was in my early experiences that I learned that church people are people. Period. I made it my business to be kind to newcomers so that they would not experience what I did, a least not from me.

I had been in the church for some time and had never accepted Christ as Lord and Savior, which I think was just overlooked by most people. After several months, a brother in the church caught me after service and asked, "Did I accept Jesus Christ as my Lord and Savior?" I hesitantly replied, "No," because I was afraid of what I had to do. He assured me it was simple, and all I had to do is repeat after him. I did, and it was that simple; I repeated after him, believed, and I was saved. That is why, as a leader in the church I made it my business to do an altar call at the end of every service. Every experience is an opportunity for us to learn what to do and even what not to do.

Despite being in the church, the truth is I would still go to parties on Friday nights, hang out on Saturday nights, and then go to church on Sunday. I'll never forget one of my significant testimonies. I remember feeling weird one day when I was at a club with my friends, and we were there dancing and carrying on, having a ball. I was 18 years old at the time. There were mirrors all around the club, and then I remember that the mirrors got really foggy. I begin to feel really weird, and in my spirit, I remember a small voice saying, "You don't belong here." I knew it was God because I didn't (and don't) drink, nor did I smoke. Before salvation, I wanted to be like my mom who always told me all of her friends drink and smoke but she never did. She always said, "I never follow the crowd." Although I tried to drink and couldn't stand the taste of alcohol, I also couldn't stand the smell of tobacco.

Now when my friends were smoking weed, I didn't mind smelling that; however, that one experience with my aunt letting me inhale a cigarette because I was begging, almost choking me to death when I was younger convinced me that I never wanted to smoke in life again. Mission accomplished, Auntie.

So, I knew I wasn't high, but I just couldn't shake that feeling. I went to my girlfriend and told her that I needed to go. I just remember being pressed to leave and getting home at maybe 2 or 3 o'clock in the morning. I just wanted to rest and get to church the next Sunday.

Well, on that Monday, we got a call and learned that two of our girlfriends were in a shoot-out at the club. One girlfriend was grazed on her face, as a matter of fact, the bullet just missed going through her head. Another friend got shot in her leg. I was blown away and saying to myself, "Oh my goodness, God really spoke to me and had me leave." Who knows where I would have gotten shot or if I would have survived for that matter?

I heard people telling stories about God, I listened to the speeches about miracles and the miraculous and all of that, but at that point, something triggered within me. God spared my life. From that point forward, I got serious about the things of God. I decided that I was done going to clubs. I began to really, really get involved in my church. I was so faithful--never missing a service. And back then, we had Sunday morning service, Sunday evening service, Tuesday night service, and Friday night service. Then we would go out witnessing and evangelizing on Saturdays, and there was choir rehearsal on Mondays. I was basically in church all week, to the point that my mom was annoyed because I was never home, and when I was there, I was coming back late.

I became so involved so fast to the point where it seemed that my girlfriends that were coming to the church were starting to fall off. They weren't coming as much as I was, and when I tried to get them to, they were like, "Oh no, we are young and have a life outside of this." So, once I decided I was going to be set apart, they started to fall back. One day one of the prayer warriors was preaching, and she called me out to tell me that I was set apart and called out from amongst them. This happened while my friends were still in the church. Then when they started to fall off, I thought about the message and that word, and I became okay with it.

My friends kept saying that there was something different about me, and I felt that I was where I was supposed to be. I even gave up my boyfriend at the time when I first came to church.

People knew he was special because I used to put his name on my ring fingernail and wear it to church. He was that favorite boyfriend I spoke of earlier. I had to tell him that as a Christian, there are just some things we can't do anymore. He didn't understand, and he also couldn't relate to this new life of mine. I told him he should consider coming to church, and I invited him to join me, but he didn't want to make such a drastic change or choice at the time. When I look back, I do understand. I was new in my relationship with Christ and I was struggling to grasp and explain this change in my life. Plus, I was also young. I told him that we didn't need to be together anymore, which upset him. He did plead his case, but after a while, he gave up. A few months later, he surprised me and popped up to my church. He was like, "Oh, I want to get back with you, and I'll change. I'll come to church."

At this point, it was too late. The pastor's son and I had already started something being that we weren't really cousins. He began letting me know that he was attracted to me and how I'd grown up so beautifully. I had become a part of a new culture, and although that last boyfriend was good, he didn't understand where I was and where I was going. So, I declined.

Suddenly, the pastor's son/my cousin/ "framily" and I are having not just a relationship, but a sexual relationship. I don't know when it started, but all I know is that I started hanging out at his house in between services, and he began to get a little close. I remember feeling really good, because I think I was always secretly crushing on him. I just didn't always feel like it was the right thing to do being that we were in the church. But, I was the babe in Christ and I had just come from this behavior. He always knew what to say and what to do, to get me right where he wanted me. Even if I said, "We shouldn't be doing this," that never changed anything.

The only problem was we were heavily in church, and every now and again, the word would convict us, or me. After hearing the word and I knew it was wrong, but once you are caught up, it's just not that easy to stop.

I remember hearing the Word of God after being with him and feeling bad all the time. I was a member of the choir and also leading praise and worship; he's the pastor's son and organist, and here we are in sin. We would hang out with other young people on the weekends, but we would always find time to sneak away and hook up. I remember it being uncomfortable if somebody preached about sin. So, after a while, I just wanted to get married. This is the church person's way of wanting to have guilt-free sex. I know many young people in the church who got married, and it didn't last because they just wanted to have guilt-free sex.

I was unable to see and admit this then, but I see now that the problem with marrying this man was that we were not in a real relationship. We would go together for a couple weeks, then we would break up, and he would have another person he was dating. They would date for a little while and then break up, and he would come back to me. I remember being hurt so many times.

At the same time, my self-esteem is chipping away, because some of the girls he was dating were light-skinned, and you know my issues with that. If I cut my hair, he would tell me I need to let my hair grow longer. If I cut down my nails, he would ask me to let them grow or do certain things with my nails. All the while, there were getting back "togethers" and breakups. Because of our involvement in church, I'm with him five or six days a week, whether we go together or not. If I lead worship, I have to communicate with him, the organist. We are still in this gospel rap group together. I write all the hooks and sing them. And we get invited to concerts and other events all the time where I witness him flirting with other women. I'm also competing for his attention with the woman in the church that like him as well. He was such a flirt, and I didn't even realize that I was being completely disrespected the entire time. My silly, uninformed self would then say, "Well, I'm going to pray, because maybe he's not ready now, but if I pray, he will mature and one day realize all that we've been through, and he'll come back and marry me." I had this stupid fairytale dream of him realizing that because I'm a singer and he's an organist, and we both have a special call on our lives, he'll realize that I am his wife.

It was stupid, but over my years of research and counseling women, this is the sad mistake a lot of women in the church have made. Wasting their lives, while a man is showing you who they are, but secretly waiting for them. Why believe God for what I already have--a toxic relationship?!

I wanted to be with him for all of the wrong reasons. He was tall, dark, and handsome; he had the swag I was attracted to, and he was driving a nice car. He was great for my image. Walking in a room with him was awesome. All eyes on us. We made a beautiful couple (if only I knew then I was beautiful all by myself).

Then I had the 'we grew up' together story, but the truth is we weren't that close growing up. I had created a fantasy in my head. I never considered that we didn't really ever 'date-date.' All we did was go to church and hang out at the house afterward, go back to church, and hang out with friends at times. If we were honest, at that age, we didn't even know who we were or what we wanted.

He was always struggling with trying to get approval and attention from his dad. That's a whole other story. He didn't have the relationship he wanted with his dad, and he was really sour about that, so a lot of times, I think that's why he kept messing around with all the women. He would get in trouble for those things but not in trouble enough. But, it was enough to get the attention of his dad. I believe this all contributed towards the reason why he behaved the way he behaved. He had also seen this behavior in church. So getting in trouble never stopped him. Despite being the organist and in a very visible ministry role, there were never any real consequences for his behavior.

But that didn't really matter to me. As a young lady, I needed the kind of guidance that would have helped me to understand I didn't have to accept this treatment. The relationship would be so on and off, but I was so in love with him that whenever he wanted me, I would come back. I was so busy loving him, but I wasn't loving myself.

I could feel his presence at times, and he would call me, and I would just run back into his arms.

He would give me a look when I was mad at him at church, and it was on after church. I continued to set myself up by having my seat in the front on the organ side so that I could keep his attention. All the while, I was totally not around my family anymore. I was being taught that when you get saved, you can't hang with everybody; you can't go to family events because it's carnal. In all my faithfulness, I became one of the primary praise and worship leaders, and later, a Junior Missionary. After being completely committed and faithful to the choir, I was a choir director and then the vice president of the choir. Then I became a Missionary and then an evangelist, where I preached my first trial sermon. After an increase in my prayer life and leading praise and worship, I was being told there was an anointing on my life. That is a gift and enablement to minister effectively in service. I never asked for any of those titles or positions; they were given to me according to my faithfulness. I know a lot of people testify that they felt the call on their life and put in the work for their titles. I have had many titles in 25 years of ministry, and I can tell you I never asked for one of them. As a matter of fact, every time I got one, it scared the hell right out of me.

I will say this, though. I remember being a teenager and hearing a woman preacher who sang so powerfully and then preached an awesome word. There was something that ignited in my spirit, and I said, "If that is what my ministry would look like, and can make such an impact, I don't mind it." It was scary to me then, and to this day, I'm still afraid to grace the pulpit to give the word. I don't want to be responsible for steering God's people the wrong way or messing anyone up. Over the years, many prophets and many men and women of God have come in and confirmed the call on my life. I also knew that whenever I sang, preached, or even just led sessions with youth, women, and small groups, there was great fulfillment in seeing God's people blessed. Even when I choreographed for the youth dance ministries at my church, that was fulfilling. I loved going to the nursing homes and the prisons, seeing people's hearts filled. If that means that I am called, I'll do it for the rest of my days. With all of that, I was still battling in this toxic relationship.

After three years of the crap, from 17 to 20 years old (*Lord, I was still a baby! Where was the guidance?),* I decided I didn't want to go through this anymore. Furthermore, he brought a girl to the church who was a couple years younger than me, and he dated her for longer than a couple weeks. I remember feeling afraid that this could be serious because it was lasting longer than the others. The nail in the coffin was when we were broken up, and he picked me up with her in the car. That was it. I had enough.

I met a new guy through a mutual friend. He was really cool, and he adored me. He was like, "Oh my God, you're so beautiful; I want to make you my first lady one day." I was trying to get this guy to take it slow. I explained to him that I had just gotten out of a relationship, but he still offered to take me out. I explained that I was probably still in love, but if he's okay with that, we could see what happens.

One day my date came to pick me up from church. Service had not quite ended, and he (the pastor's son, my 'ex') saw that I got up to leave and was outraged. I think he knew at this point that I was dating someone. He jumped off the organ and followed me out to the rotunda. He demanded to know where I was going and with who. Angrily, I let him know that it was none of his business. Well, to make a long story short, shortly after a couple of dates, he dropped that other girl with the quickness, and he told me he loved me, and he wanted me to be his wife. He started spitting the same words I've been crying out for over the past of couple years; saying that we had been through too much together and we were meant to be.

Well, I felt as though my prayers had been answered, and I dropped that poor new guy so fast! Seriously though, I did tell him that my heart was somewhere else. I never really gave that relationship a chance because I never got over the last.

I was so happy. My dream (which was really the beginning of a nightmare) was finally coming true. I felt as though my prayers were answered. This is when I found out that *God will allow you to get what you want, even if it's not good for you.* I did have one or two people who told me to be careful. One of the ministers said, «You may be good for him, but he may not be good for you.» Lord, I wish I would›ve listened! We immediately began to put together a nice little wedding at the church. All of the workers were so glad to be a part of the committee planning the pastor›s son›s wedding. Mind you, at the time I am 20 and he is 22 years old. We were kids about to dabble in grown folks› business.

Chapter 5

FIRST MARRIAGE: CONFIDENCE BROKEN

It's the end of summer 1997. I am 20 years old and I am planning a wedding. I didn't finish college because I got so involved in church, and that took over my life. I didn't care because ministry was so important to me, and that was my idea of putting God first. I started John Jay College right after I graduated from high school; thinking that I wanted to be a lawyer. I did really well the first semester and I withdrew from classes the second semester. At that point, I decided to give God my whole life. I did just that, being in church nearly 7 days a week. I was working at Kelly's Temp Agency at the time, doing receptionist and data entry jobs.

See, I started coming in very late from church all the time. My mom was beginning to question why I had to be in church all the time, and why I was coming in so late. Well, if you work with the Bishop, or are family of the Bishop, the men usually stay with him after service while he's counseling and doing whatever he does in the office. Those who ride with the men have to wait with them, which would be very late most of the time, way after midnight. Then someone carries his things and his briefcase to his car and sees him off. In this culture, this is called covering the man of God. The people covering him are called the adjutants.

As I said, I was getting home very late, at 17 and 18 years old. My mother couldn't understand why the church is taking all night and why I had to be there every day. I begin to challenge her, reminding her that it was her idea for me to go to church. She then took my keys and started locking me out. At that point, I decided that since I finally started going to church and was all in, I wasn't going to let her stop me. My God-sister was getting sick of her parents as well, so we decided to get an apartment in Canarsie, while I was working a job at Sears. Unfortunately, they cut my hours at Sears and I couldn't pay my rent, which got me locked out of that apartment. My God-sister didn't want to jeopardize her stay there, so she had to comply. She was good because her parents were helping her with her rent and almost everything else. I started realizing that adulting is no fun, toilet paper just doesn't walk in the house, I had to buy everything that I needed myself. My money wasn't adding up. Now I understood what my mother meant about money, not growing on trees.

Now I'm locked out of my apartment, and my God sister is afraid to let me in. A couple of the ministers helped me break into my apartment and get the furniture that my grandmother so lovingly bought for me. Then I moved in with my best friend, who lived with her Gomer (creole for grandma). Their rent was very low, so it worked out for me. My best friend and I found jobs as telemarketers trying to sell home security. I sold everybody in my family and at my church a security system! After only working there for a few months, that job went out of business and that's when I decided to work for a temp agency.

While planning this wedding, everybody bought everything for us. My grandmother bought my gown; I think his dad paid for the flowers, decorations, and wedding ring. They got a committee together to put it all together and make it work. I called my best friend from high school and some of the ladies in the church to be in my bridal party. Meanwhile, he is getting his boys and cousins to be in the wedding also.

When he asked to marry me, we also agreed not to have sex before the wedding day to make it special. A few days before the wedding, he got the itch and wanted to. I nicely reminded him of our agreement, but he got very upset and threatened to call off the wedding if I didn't do it. I remember thinking he was joking until he started to call my best friend at the time to tell her we were calling it off. I started crying and begging him not to do that. My grown-up self is ashamed and embarrassed to say I went through with it. I was shocked that he couldn't wait just a couple of days for the wedding day. That was so childish, and deep down inside, I knew we shouldn't get married. That scenario also may have been him trying to get out, knowing he wasn't ready. I should've let him call it off. The whole immature scene proves that we were not ready to be married. We were just kids.

Meanwhile, a young lady that he met at one of the shows we had done that he invited to the church goes to the office and tells the Bishop that he cannot marry me because the

Lord said that he was her husband. This was the stuff I had to go through being with this guy. His dad told me don't worry about it, she's fantasizing it's nothing. Do you know the same young lady came in with sunglasses on crying to my wedding? These are the crazy things that happen in church.

It was a beautiful wedding, and we were a beautiful couple. When asked is there anyone that objects to this wedding, this idiot holds his mouth as if he was going to say something, scaring the crap out of me, only to turn around give up his black book to his best friend. My uncles were getting ready to get up and hurt him. To this day, I still don't find that funny.

Now, I know that getting married at this age was probably the dumbest thing we could've ever done. I didn't have a life plan for myself. I don't think he had a life plan either. And we surely didn't have a life plan together. We were married in October, and his dad decided he was going to pay our rent for the rest of the year. I guess this was an extended wedding gift. He did have a job, and I think he was paying the utilities in the apartment. I believe that we took over an apartment that his aunt had been living in. Still, I knew that my temp agency positions weren't consistent enough, and we had to prepare to take over the bills.

My grandmother assisted me in getting a job at the New York City Department of Education as a teacher's aide. She was a UFT (union) representative and a reading teacher, so she was able to get me hired pretty quickly. I started out as a substitute teacher in a special education class in April and then became permanent by the new school year.

Not even sixty days in, the marriage devastation begins. My then husband started going on and on about how he had made a mistake marrying me. You can't imagine how utterly hurt and devastated I was. I was already overwhelmed by the responsibilities of being his wife because he was so picky and finicky about everything. His shirts had to be a turned all a certain way, all the brushes had to be aligned in a specific way, and God forbid you lose anything! It was indeed turning into a nightmare. Additionally, because we had to maintain a particular image as the pastor's family, you'd better have yourself together and look perfect also.

So, honestly, I don't even remember having happy days with this man, and then BAM-two months later, he's saying this was all a mistake. He was also telling me he was in love with the girl that he was with previously. The only thing I could think is, "How could you or why would you marry me, if you still loved her? As a matter of fact, you were with her but you came back to me." I just remember feeling as though my heart was shattered. I waited so long to have this, and now it was being taken away from me.

There were so many issues I can't even name them all. So, the 2nd, then 3rd, and 4th months, I found myself genuinely hanging on to my marriage by a thread. Of course, it was all me. I was reading every marriage book I could get my hands on, I was attending every women's meeting, and I was asking him repeatedly, "What can we do to fix this?" But nothing was working. He would go out and come in late. He would sometimes stay out all night. Then, he would get home for church, and I had to ride with him. Sometimes I would get up to sing, and they would announce me, and being married, we had the same last name. After announcing me, he would say, "She's not Mrs. So-and-so anymore" in front of the congregation. I was miserable. I can remember getting up to sing solos and being unable to make it through the song without falling on my knees crying. I remember singing with the choir and being unable to make it to the end of the song without crying. I'm not sure if this was faith, faithfulness, or pure stupidity. Because faithfulness was heavily taught, through all of it, I never missed a service, and I continued to be faithful to everything that I was a part of, including the choir where I had to deal with him. Meanwhile, he made it clear to everyone that he talked to that he did not want to be married anymore. I was living a life of embarrassment and shame.

Then around month ten, he went to a conference and came back saying he was going to try to make it work. Clearly, I was surprised but overjoyed! And again, I felt as though my prayers were being answered. He said he was at a conference with a friend (I now know the friend was another woman) and that the preacher said something profound, and it stuck with him. My husband told me that the speaker said, "You know why would you want to go with the ‹what if?› Why would you do that when God has given you everything that you need?»

I don't remember the whole speech, but all I know is that he was going to try to make it work. And for one or two months, he did. I recall him being kind and loving, and me not feeling "as" insecure. I can't say all the insecurity was gone because it didn't vanish after him making me feel insecure for years. It was so good to him; he said, "Let's have a baby." And because of this month or so of real goodness with him, I agreed, but I didn't believe it would happen so fast. But, I was now 21, we were married, and we decided to stop using condoms and then… bam! In month eleven, I realized I was pregnant.

Everything was going great, but around and shortly after our first anniversary, he started acting up again. I overheard him on the phone with a close female friend on Christmas day sharing that he had gotten his mom a beautiful Anne Klein watch for Christmas, but he had only gotten me some barrettes. He was laughing and thought that this was so funny. I was outraged. I cursed him out, with choice words that I won't say now. I had never spoken to him in this manner because I never wanted to jeopardize our relationship. I guess my hormones were raging, being four months pregnant, and I just wasn't having it. After the argument, he left. He left me there by myself on Christmas Day. In past years, even when we weren't married, we house hopped on Christmas together. I had no car and no money, but thankfully one of my girlfriends came and got me so I wouldn't be alone. She called me because she was the pastor's sister-in-law, and when he got to her house, she asked where I was. She was concerned, and after he left, she called me and came to get me. I packed up a week's worth of clothes and hung out with her for the week. Thankfully, they cheered me up.

When I got back home after that week, I felt better, and I was going to continue to believe God for my marriage. My husband came in with one of his protégés that he was teaching to play the organ and started packing up all his things. The young guy looked so confused and concerned for me. He asked if I was okay, and I told him that I wasn't, but I was going to be. My husband looked at me and said, "I realized that while you were gone that week that I could live without you, so I'm leaving." I don't think anyone could ever understand the way my heart dropped and how my stomach began to feel queasy. I didn't know what to say nor do. That young man, his protégé, had loved me so much, we had become like his family. I could even see the pain in his eyes, so I tried to fix my face and suck it up, to ease his concern.

I later found out that my husband had moved back in with his grandmother. I was devastated because working as a teacher's aide and maybe making $14,000 a year; I knew that I couldn't live in our apartment much longer. One of my friends from church needed an apartment and could not afford a place by herself, so we began to live together. She had a son and a newborn. That newborn laid in my bed on my stomach every night while I was pregnant. She was a good roommate; she bought the groceries, I cooked, we shared utilities with no problem. We cleaned up together, loved the same music, and went to church together. We lived there for months. I was still dealing with my baby daddy, being a complete idiot telling people the marriage is over even though I was pregnant, and we were not yet divorced. And again, I remained faithful to everything that I did in my church. He started to bring this girl back to church while I was pregnant. I asked if this was even okay. I can't remember exactly, but I think his father stepped up and said that this would not be okay.

He wanted to make it known that this was the girl who he really wanted to be with, and he did. My grandmother and

I didn't live too far from each other, so she would come over to look out for me. One day she overheard that I had the girl's number and decided to call her. Her mother answered the phone. My grandmother said, "Your daughter is messing with a married man who has a pregnant wife." Her mother's reply was, "He doesn't really love your granddaughter; he really loves my daughter. He was with her first and loved her first." My grandmother then said, "You have your stories mixed up because these two grew up together, and my granddaughter had been with him for several years before your daughter even met him." I remember having this conversation with the young lady as well when they were dating the first time. I told her, "You got yourself mixed up in an ongoing relationship, and you might not want to get mixed up in this, because he leaves them all and comes back to me." This was true, but I was stuck with all that he was when I got him back. I should have let all those women have him.

I worked my entire pregnancy with special education children who sometimes fought and cussed me out, students with ADHD, students with so many emotional issues. As my pregnancy was ending, I had a couple of baby showers, one with my family and one with the church. I got so much stuff. People really loved me (and him for that matter), so they showered us with many gifts.

This was going to be the pastor's first grandchild. And still, the entire time, this man is trying to get me to sign divorce papers. How cruel was that: carrying his child and he's trying to get me to sign divorce papers?

The Day I Committed Suicide

But no matter how many times he would try to force me to sign divorce papers, I was determined that my child was not going to be born a bastard, so he would just have to wait. This only caused him to be even more rude, mean, and belligerent. It was tough. I remember crying a lot and being constantly embarrassed. But I kept standing, and I kept singing. And if I can be honest, I secretly hoped that if he saw our beautiful baby, he would want to make it work. After refusing a couple of times, he finally gave up and said he'll wait till after the baby was born.

I'll never forget the last week of June. I was so big; I thought I would have had the baby by now. I was creeping up on my due date.

Every year the church went away for convocation, which was the gathering of the churches of the organization that we were part of. The norm was to get plane money together to caravan, collect room money, and travel to be a part of this event. I could not go this year because I was nine months pregnant, and the baby could come at any moment. I asked my husband not to go to convocation because I felt that he should not miss the birth of our child. Well, guess what? He said, "Don't worry, I'm going to go, and I'll be back before the baby is born." I remember feeling totally hurt by this man yet again. The next night, I danced around to Whitney Houston's song, "It's not right, but it's okay." I danced so hard that I had pains in my stomach and my back. The next morning, I felt a pain in my back that I couldn't describe. I called my grandmother and said, "Listen, I have a doctor's appointment at 12, but it's 9 am, and I'm starting to feel a pain in my back every five minutes." She said, "Girl, go to your doctor's appointment now, and I'll meet you there."

When I got to my doctor's appointment, she told me that I was already 5cm dilated and that I should walk across the street to Brookdale Hospital and prepare to have this baby. She also told me I should walk around because I could get closer to 10 cm before they hooked me up to machines and would be unable to move. But, by the time I walked across the street, the pain was coming so bad that I immediately went to the doctors and asked for pain relievers. And this was after I had told everyone that I was going to have a natural birth with no medication! Before I knew it, my mom, my sister, my cousin my aunt, his mom, and some of the godparents were all up there, as I was in labor for about nine hours. The epidural was working so well I was giggling and laughing, and when it wore off I asked for more. Well, nine hours later and after four re-ups of epidural, they had to break my water because I was 10 cm and my water hadn't broken. And still, there were no signs of my husband/baby daddy.

After they broke my water, they refused to give me any more epidural because they said it was time for the baby to come. They had me push a few times with my mom holding one hand and his mom holding the other. Once they saw the head with all that hair on it, they wheeled me into the labor room and asked who was coming with me. I said, "Definitely, my mother." 2,3,4 pushes later, and my baby girl, my firstborn, was born June 23, 1999, at nine something p.m. While I was in labor, everyone was at convocation trying to find a way to get her father back to see her birth. He finally made it as I was rolling out of the delivery room, and I just stared at him in disgust. I really didn't have anything to say to him because I was very disappointed. He was horrible to me, but the least that he could have committed to was seeing her born.

My dad came up the next day and saw us. He was so happy to be a grandpa. My family was with me in the hospital for two days until they put me out. If you and the baby are healthy, they waste no time putting you out of the hospital.

I had my daughter in June, and as a teaching assistant, I had the rest of the summer off with pay. Once September rolled in, I had to go back to work, and my grandmother, who was retired, decided that she would keep my baby for me while I was at work. She didn't live too far from me, and she didn't mind taking the bus to get to me in the mornings. It was nice but short-lived because my roommate did get married and move out.

My roommate met a guy, and they were getting really close. This is a funny story. She met the guy and gave him our number, but when he called, my voice and name were on the answering machine. He said to himself, "I know this girl, and there can only be one Janelka." Well, come to find out, this guy that she met was someone that attended the same junior high school. They got really close and were planning to get married.

Well, when she got married, I could not afford to stay in the place I was living, so I ended up moving into one of the rooms at my husband's grandmother's house, ...which was the same house where he lived. Now at this point, I had to watch him bring other women in and out while I was pregnant, including the girl he supposedly was going back to/leaving me for. On top of that, he was still wanting and trying to sleep with me as well.

In the midst of it all, every Sunday I would go to church. As a matter of fact, my baby was only two weeks old when I brought her out for the tent revival. I did get cussed out by the mother's board, for having my baby outside for the revival, but the excitement of those two weeks changed my baby sleep pattern, and she had been sleeping, from around 9–10 pm to 8 am ever since.

So now I'm "single-momming" it to church, to work, and back home. One of her godmothers would babysit her during the day, as she had started a small daycare center. The hard thing was that I would travel on the bus with the baby and her chair to drop her off and to go to work and after picking her up. I remember it being so hard. On top of that, he was really pressing me for this divorce again.

Sometimes when I had a solo at church, they would mention me by name, and he would get angry and yell out that that was not my name, although we weren't divorced yet. He was so mean to me, and I was still sitting in the front while all of these people were watching my life fall apart. He was still adamantly trying to divorce me because he was determined to be with the girl he was with before we got married. The white Honda Accord that I had purchased wound up being a lemon after my grandmother gave me $1000 to get it. It only lasted a few months before we found out the engine was bad.

This was why I was traveling on the train and bus everywhere. Then I got a red Hyundai Elantra. That little red car got me a few places with my daughter. I don't remember what happened to that car, but I do remember my last hoopty: a blue Ford aspire.

My husband at the time was adamant about getting a divorce, and so he kept trying to get me to sign the papers. I finally decided to stop taking this emotional abuse and accepted that it was over. I decided that I was going to allow myself to be free from this torture. This was the most embarrassing devastating hurtful thing that I could ever go through, and I went through it publicly—in front of everyone in my church.

When I read the papers, it somehow said that I had abandoned him. Then he wanted to have joint custody of our daughter. I told him I would not be signing these papers because I did nothing to him and that he was the one cheating on me and mistreating me. I also said since he wanted out of the marriage, I wanted to have full custody of our daughter. I really didn't know what everything in the divorce papers meant, but I knew that it didn't say the right thing and that it wasn't in my favor. And there was no way I was going to allow him to treat me the way that he did and have the divorce papers stating that I was the problem. He was so mad because he had to draw up the papers more than once, which was costing him more and more money. I didn't care, and when it said what it was supposed to say, I gracefully signed.

I was determined to get my life back on track. I was on the altar, praying just to get my mind back and for my heart to be right. I can remember driving over the bridge one time and thinking that my life was over and wanting to drive right off. Another time I was driving and tried to imagine what would happen if I just ran into the pole. But, I knew that my daughter needed me, and I chose to live. I declared that I shall live and not die; that I was here to declare the works of the Lord.

I became a youth minister, a junior missionary, and preached in my trial sermon at this time because I was sold out and committed to God. My prayer life and relationship with God increased during this time. I even thought about moving to the South where my uncle lived, but during my time of prayer, and counsel with a few people, we thought it would best to cultivate what God is doing in my life here. Although I believe everything happens for a reason, and it's all working together for my good, I don't think it was the wisest thing to stay there and watch him get back with this girl and actually marry her right in my face. There were so many churches in Brooklyn that I didn't have to stay there and experience further embarrassment. Looking back, I realize people will counsel you to do what they think is best; to do that which is beneficial to them. However, it is important to have a relationship with God for yourself, along with knowledge, education, and common sense. There was absolutely no reason that I should have stayed in that environment.

I no longer wanted to hang out with the young people in my circle anymore. My spiritual life had intensified, so I started hanging out with a different crew. I began hanging out with the older saints, and those that were praying on the altar. My prayer life increased in pursuit of rebuilding my life. I realized that as a single mother, I didn't want to make such a small salary.

I moved around in District 17 in the New York City Department of Education, working with a lot of youth. Because I was young and always looked close to their age, they took to me. They came from very impoverished and gang-infested communities. I found myself counseling even though I was just a teacher's assistant. I decided to go back and get my degree, majoring in psychology, in pursuit of becoming a school counselor. I went to the College of New Rochelle Brooklyn campus, which worked for students who were working and needed to maximize the time while maximizing the credits per semester. The more education I had, the more money I could make as well, so this worked for me. I was on my way to rebuilding my life, and things were looking pretty good.

This was many years ago and I must acknowledge that after a few years of tension and conflict, co-parenting has been very pleasant and he is a great father to my oldest daughter to this day.

Chapter 6

SECOND MARRIAGE: REBUILDING CONFIDENCE

This chapter is extremely important to me because if there was one lesson that I learned, it's that you need to be completely and totally healed before moving on into a new relationship. The truth is that a lot of people, especially women, who are hurt, think that they want a good man. However, when you are not healed after exiting a toxic and unhealthy relationship, what you really end up looking for is a paramedic. A paramedic is a first responder that shows up, takes your vitals, and keeps you stable before the more qualified medical staff with the more powerful, hospital-grade equipment can attend to your health crisis. Well, in the same way, when people exit an unhealthy relationship, what they often seek is a new one, when what they need to do is take their time to become whole before entering a new relationship.

After my first marriage, I became good friends with my second husband. He had also been going through a divorce, so we had that in common. However, he was different from all of us because he was so super religious even though he was young; I always thought he was a lot older than me because he acted old. Truthfully, I still wonder how we became close because he was so churchy, and his characteristics were not something that I ordinarily would have been attracted to. Additionally, he was always sending everyone to hell! He was continually telling the youth, especially, "If you're doing this, you're going to hell" and "If you do that, then you are going to hell." It was so annoying because no one was safe from the "prophet." I remember shortly after meeting him (and not even knowing him that well) he tried to tell me that if I stopped messing with my ex he would marry me. I checked him quickly told him he was off and that he needed to mind his business. I know now he was exercising his prophetic gift on everyone trying to sharpen it. I wasn't with it though and told him he didn't know what he was talking about. Remember, I wasn't that saved yet.

It was at that point where he was telling everybody that we had to call him "Prophet," and I recall not liking him at all. First, I thought he was an arrogant know-it-all and he acted like an old man. I was shocked when I found out he was only about four years older than me. Yet, everything changed when he went through his divorce. It humbled him. I believe any time you get divorced in church it has an impact on you because you end up feeling judged. This humbled him because now he was the sinner and wasn't sending anyone to hell anymore.

So, I started hanging out with the sanctified, praying, and preaching crowd. A couple of us had been divorced. I stayed on the altar. Being that I was no longer with my first husband and sometimes in between cars, I would get rides from friends. He would drive me at times. I told him this was a good place for him and that the reason everyone was talking about him and pointing a finger was that he was so hard on them. But this made him nicer, and I decided to have compassion toward him even when others didn't.

You can always tell when someone is trying to get close. He was offering to drive me home more and more, and eventually, he was taking me home more than anyone else. At this time, I was living with my ex-husband's grandmother. In fact, my ex-husband had just remarried in my face, and it devastated me.

Again, that is why it is so important to be healed. Soon, I found myself talking to this guy from church more and more. There was this time he had to preach in California or somewhere, and I told him to call me, and he did. I think he was comfortable with me because he felt a level of acceptance. He was comfortable, and I also was feeling a level of acceptance and friendship right after my ex-husband just killed my self-esteem by constantly telling me that I was not pretty enough, my hair wasn't long enough, my skin was not light enough, and so on! He talked a lot about my ministry and how awesome I would be in ministry with him.

Now, this guy is taking me to nice dinners, being super cool and nice to me, and so this relationship started moving at a rapid rate. The conversation of sex comes up, and we are both young, and the flesh was heavy. He is still very religious, and now he is saying things to me like, "I see the call of God on your life, and for where we are going, there is no reason for us to live in sin." He saw us doing ministry together. I didn't want to be in sin and having a prayer life; I had my convictions. We felt compatible and saw a future. I do remember there being doubt on both our hearts. I did mention that if we weren't going to be together, I would just move down South as I had initially planned to do after my marriage was over. There was too much here that had happened that I would like to get away from and start fresh.

Our friendship was great, and we cared for each other, but we were hot and young in lust. I may not have been that experienced, but I did like sex. This is another church culture thing: instead of trying to be celibate, we used the scripture, "it's better to marry than to burn." Boy, were we naïve. So here I am almost two years out of my last marriage at 25 years old getting married again.

We quietly got married because of my ex-husband and his family. Both of our exes were still members of the church, so we wanted to spare the drama. I don›t know why we were trying to be secretive, and now I am not sure why we were sparing my ex-husband›s feelings because he had forced me to sign divorce papers, was openly mean to me in public and got married without asking or sparing my feelings. Eventually, a few weeks later, we told everyone. If we were going to choose to be together, we should have left and started fresh.

When my first husband got married to the other woman being that the church we were attending was his dad's church, I should have left. But we were taught to stay faithful, loyal, and to be at every service. We were also taught that when God places you somewhere, if you leave, you lose your call, your blessing, and the leader that God put over your life. I was too young and impressionable to know better. Now, when I remarried, that should have been a time to leave and start fresh again, but "nooooo", we stayed, and all did ministry together. In looking back at that time, there was no premarital counseling either time nor was there any counseling after either of us went through our divorce. And trust me- we both needed it. We needed to funnel through the pain, our decisions, our faults, and all the effects of a failed marriage.

Things were going well. After being in a tiny one-bedroom for less than a year, the landlord's parents had a five-bedroom home they wanted to rent out after leaving to retire south. My husband's gift of negotiating always worked in his favor, and we ended up renting for very little. It was perfect: we already had three kids; I had my girl and his two boys would come over for weekends and I felt like that was perfect for us. We didn't even need any more kids, yet one day we were prophesized to that we would have five kids. After I gave the confused and disappointed look the prophet said, that we would have all the help that we needed. Honestly, we used to get prosperity prophecies all of the time. But I still wasn't thinking about having five kids.

Then, things started changing a bit. I remember being in the kitchen, and he came in and said, "Hmm, from the way you are stirring that pot, it doesn't look like you know what you are doing. You can't cook." At the time, in my twenties, I couldn't cook the way I can now, but I just remember being very intimidated at that moment because I had heard stories of how the women in his family were from the south, and they used to throw down in the kitchen. My first husband was ok with the simple meals that I cooked. So, after that, I barely wanted to cook for him at all. If I'm going to be judged before the meal was even cooked, why bother? I didn't take rejection well, but hell, if you don't have a fighting chance, how should you proceed?

He took me shopping so I could look like the prosperous couple we were becoming. He told me I should try wearing make-up. I asked, "Why? Am I not pretty enough?" He said, "Yes, but it's like the clothes of your face. It enhances it." So, I started to look at magazines, and I liked wearing and playing with a little make-up. I began to conform to his wants and needs, and I didn't see anything wrong with it because we are to do the things that make our spouses happy. Plus, this was our second marriage, so we can't fail again.

Then the next thing that came up was him talking to me about the affair that led to the divorce in his first marriage. He cheated on his wife with someone who was very experienced. Although I loved being intimate, I still wasn't very experienced. Therefore, after hearing the tricks she had done, in order to figure out how to please him I decided that I would have to watch some pornography in order to learn how to do the things that he was describing that he wanted. What I learned is if you have preferences, especially in the bedroom, it's ok to say what you want, but don't use a person that you had it with to express that. I was now feeling intimidated by someone he may have still had access to. That is not something you want to do to your spouse.

While dealing with the challenges of newlywed life, I was also still having trouble with my ex-husband. Though I had my feelings about it, allowing him to take his daughter with his new wife, worked out because it gave us a break sometimes. He was impossible to co-parent with at times, and he didn't want to pay child support because he was mad that I remarried. He thought I was going just to be lonely on the side while he went and got happily married. There was someone he looked up to that got married but had an ex around him who would do anything for him. This woman was still in love with that man, and he kept her around. When my ex and I were breaking up, he said I was going to be that woman to him. What a jerk!

I don't want to even touch the dysfunction and disrespect in that situation. That's another book entirely, but it goes on a lot in the church and needs to be addressed and dealt with, especially when the leaders are the ones facilitating the dysfunction and disrespect. Woman are in awe with these men in power, and they are shamefully using this (godly) power (which is really their insecurities) to cultivate these dysfunctional relationships, while they are married. My ex used to say, "If you get a man, he's going to have to understand our relationship." At the time, I was strong when it was finally over, and I said, "Oh, hell no, your loss. You better go have a special relationship with the woman you chose." That's the attitude I gave him, especially when I got a new man. No access at all, just short conversations when he needed to get his daughter; he was cut off.

I don't know if it was a year after I was married, but there was this witnessing thing for the church we were doing in Harlem. Everyone was already telling me how good I looked after the free tummy tuck I received from my brother hurting his arm in my garage so badly it had to be stitch by a plastic surgeon. I was in the right place at the right time to receive that blessing. I was feeling great. I don't know what we were witnessing for now, but a few of us from the church were out in Manhattan. We took the train out there. A few weeks prior, my ex- called to check up on me knowing my husband had left me home during a blackout right after my surgery. I think they announced in the church.

While on the train, my ex starts reminiscing about our rap group and old times. He was giving me accolades on my singing, my new look, my beauty, amongst other things. I'm not entirely sure, but I think that's when he revealed to me that he missed me. Man, I was utterly appalled. But if I can be honest, I was upset because why would you miss me now that I'm married? Why would you now have so much good to say now? When I was begging you to work on our marriage, where was all of this nostalgia?

So, I tried to ignore the fact that he had me thinking. The first feeling was knowing that I wasn't so bad. Regardless of your confidence level, if the person you're in love with and/or married to tells you all negative things about yourself, it eats away at your self-esteem and self-worth. You are left in mental anguish, wondering what's wrong with you. When a marriage fails, you feel like a failure. Sometimes you want so very bad for that person to see and to know that you are worthy, beautiful, and that you are good. That is why sometimes we try to show our exes how good we are doing when we move on. But more than anything you want to make them eat their words. However, if we are honest with ourselves, we want them to validate us and to give us back our self-worth and self-esteem. It reassuring when others tell you, it's best when you know for yourself, but there's something about the moment when the person who snatched it that now wants to give it back. That's why we so desperately want them to see it. But, be careful with that! It doesn't have to come from the person who hurt you. I've learned and matured enough to know now that you can get it back with or without them. When you know it, you exude it, and then the right person sees it, falls in love with it, and will continue to nurture it.

Well, baby daddy was on a roll; the door was open, and he knew it. He would call my cell to check up on me. I hate to admit it, but at that time, I needed to hear that I was the best thing that happened to him. He was telling me everything I wanted to hear when we were married. Why now? He just knew that he messed up and wanted the chance to make it up.

He even showed up at my job, telling me he was sorry that he let me get away. He was begging me to leave my marriage so he could have his family back. So now I am feeling crazy, because I started thinking maybe I shouldn't have moved so fast. But then I remembered that he forced the divorced and remarried first. Now he sees my worth? His wife doesn't matter to me because she took him from me with no problem. At 26, with no real guidance, I didn't know what to do. What I did know is I loved knowing and feeling that he was sorry and that he finally realized my worth. He made it seem like that girl was better than me, and now it is confirmed by this that she's not. This was such a mess in every way. I was confused and torn. My husband now was an "ok" husband, but I wasn't sure; my ex was a horrible husband, but willing to make up for what he'd done and now knows what he had. What was a girl to do?

Baby daddy was my crush, and I thought life was over when he left me. He was ultimately my type tall, dark, handsome with swag, and we had a child together. Neither of us had a child with our spouses, so I wanted to go back. We were young, and we didn't give it a chance, and maybe we both moved forward too fast. We had a history as I always said, and maybe all the old prayers were finally being answered.

My husband was starting to get suspicious about me distancing myself. People started to talk. The thing that tipped me over was one day during service his wife came to me and said, "My husband said that he was going to go back to you and if you would have him back, he's leaving me. And then she asked me to please not take him back." It is a shame what I felt at that moment, but I completely felt justified in what I was feeling. I said to her, "When I pleaded with you to leave my husband alone while I was pregnant with our daughter, I was told that he didn't want me and that he was really in love with you. And you decided not to leave him alone; I don't know what to tell you." At that point, I wanted to take him back just because, I know, I was young and feeling petty, but you couldn't tell me that I wasn't justified in that.

While this is going on, my ex-husband is telling people about our long-lost love. My husband is now furious. He found out about all the talks and things that were going on with my ex-husband. I remember him punching my leg so badly in our bathroom that it left a huge bruise in my thigh.

The next argument, he was swinging a bat over my head, saying, "I should bash your head with this bat," and then it conveniently dropped out of his hand, hitting me in the head, giving me two black eyes. It was an accident, but when I told my boss that I hit the trunk of my car on my head, he didn't believe me. He thought I was being abused, and low-key slipped me information for domestic violence. I thought about it and asked myself did the bat slipped out of his hand or did he let it go. After that, I left and moved back in with my ex-husband's grandmother, and so did my ex.

Meanwhile, my husband acted as if he didn't care at first, then he came to the house, pleading for me not to do this. But I told him that he could not make me stay where I didn't want to be. I also did not like feeling torn. Don't get me wrong it wasn't right, but we as women (well, I won't speak for all women); unlike most men, we are done in our headlong before we leave, but instead of playing both sides I decided to leave. I thought it was best to go instead of my body being there and my mind elsewhere. I'm not a cheater and just couldn't do the mental back and forth. Plus, I don't want to have to lie while trying to figure it out. I'm not proud of this moment, but it is my truth.

This was crazy because now that I'm there with my ex, I realize all the hurt and pain he put me through prior. Although having our family together was a nice gesture, he was still immature, had a particular way that he wanted things to be (like his clothes all hung in the same direction, brush and comb sitting perfectly on the dresser etc.), he just wasn't super mean about it this time.

It still left a bad taste in my mouth reminding me of what a jerk he had been. He was still very image-conscious, and I realized we never really built a relationship. We always hung out with other people together, but we never talked enough to even know what we really had in common except doing music together. Our personalities pretty much clashed. I started thinking to myself, "At least my husband and I had a friendship."

So now, I was in my last semester earning my bachelor's degree, and I decided to gift myself with a brand-new car. The person I thought to go with me for a great deal was my husband. He had the gift of going into the store and talking them into deals they couldn't get themselves as the salesman. I call it the gift of gab; he was smart, charismatic, and funny. We had stopped fighting at this point. He told me he had been messing with a few girls. So, he didn't mind coming with me to help me get a good deal. He knew a lot because he was a sponge with a photogenic memory. These were all the things I liked about him.

After that deal, I felt like maybe I made a mistake. My ex was still showing all of his true colors, and I started to feel convicted about leaving. One day, I just came out and told him, "This is not ok. I can't do this anymore." I had a conversation with my ex-husband's wife, apologizing, for my intentions to hurt her like she had hurt me. I vowed if there were going to be problems with him ever again it would not have anything to do with me. I was sincerely sorry, and I realized God allowed it to end for a reason and I should have let it go. I will say this: it did bring closure in that situation for me, if nothing else. Although my ex fought me on this, with arguments and threats, it was over and I never looked back. On another note: I realize that it didn't have to go that way if I would have gotten the proper therapy and counsel needed.

At that point, I moved and found my apartment. The discussion of my husband and I getting back together was in the air. He claimed he had met someone, and it was severe, but I didn't care. I felt that we had a good thing and we were already married. I should have let it be. That would have been a good time for me to reflect on all the bad decisions made, especially in relationships up until that point. We were back and forth on the phone with his best friend of many years who became like a big sister to me. She was rooting for marriage, as most people in ministry are expected to do.

I prayed and made a vow on New Year's Eve of 2004 that if God saved our marriage, I would not get caught up again, and neither my husband nor God would have to worry about me messing up again. My husband was stubborn and filed for divorce. But then shortly after, we wound up getting back together and remarried quietly. And yet still, instead of moving on, I got stuck in the four walls of my church. It was always work, church and school. My faithfulness to God was of most importance. Plus, my church was my familiar place. What I know now is you can serve God in many ways, and in a different places. God will not penalize you for moving on. While I do believe that we are called to people, places, and things, I also believe that to stay in toxic places and situations for the sake of serving God is not God at all. I lived in Brooklyn-- there were 3 to 4 churches on almost every block. God's will and plan for your life can change locations.

When we decided to get back together, all hell broke loose. My ex and my husband began to argue and fight in the church all the time. There was always tension, and it was intense at times. My husband says that is when the Lord spoke for the second time about him stepping out to Pastor. He told me the first time he felt the Lord say to go out, and Pastor, our Bishop, said no, and said to him that he wasn't a pastor but an evangelist. He claimed to obey God and stay, but the close relationship with our Bishop and him, was never the same. He was the right hand, he ran all the teams, and he was at his house all the time and drove him everywhere, but not as much after he told him about pastoring. This time, 3 years later, he said the Lord spoke again. This time the Bishop said to him that he didn't feel it but to go ahead. This was not the sendoff he was looking for, however, it was enough for him to step out. He said that just because man doesn't feel it, doesn't mean it's not God.

We were going to go down to Georgia and start our ministry. I got excited and found new neighborhoods that were building homes in new communities for excellent prices compared to New York. Maybe this was me getting to move out of state after all. However, then a woman in Queens for whom he had been preaching for many years told him that she was about to retire and that he should start his bible study from there and see what happens. That way, when she leaves, she knows her members would be in good hands. They all loved his old school preaching and his prophetic gift. They were all six people that were left.

That was it. From April to June 2005, we had a bible study every Wednesday night. The first day we pulled in front of the church, and it was locked. He asked me if I thought that anyone was going to come. I told him that it was still early, but, "Let's go in; you got this." That day most of her people were there. The next week, they all invited someone. He used to prophesy accurately to every person there. So, they went back and invited friends to come with them every week. Each one would come back with more. We decided to make it an official church in June, opening the doors of the church, which I can't remember now but two handfuls joining, including the woman of God's members. I was the usher, the prayer warrior at the beginning of service, the praise and worship leader, and the trustee. He preached and was the sound man and sometimes helped me with praise and worship. It was a good thing I could sing acapella because I had no band. The church went from 6 people to 60 in just a few months. Our Bishop told me not to follow him, because he was not a pastor and he will probably sleep with all the women. I didn't listen because one, I made a vow about this marriage; two, the two are one, and we should not be separated; three, if that became a problem, I would deal with it when I got there like all the wives in their marriages that I had seen in ministry going through that. That's another book, but truthfully, deep down, I never felt like that would be an issue.

While doing bible study, I remained faithful to the other services at our church. It seemed like all the messages were geared to discouraging me from going with my husband. I can't stand when the messages have to be about the people in the church or somebody that makes the preacher mad. What about all the other people who came for the word? Why should they have to hear this type of message? Some things are better suited for a meeting in the office than a sermon in the pulpit.

I never disrespected authority, but there was a meeting with my ex and his dad to get me to stay. I cursed and screamed, "Listen, you brought me to this church to be saved, then screwed me (I used the F word) and played me all the way up and throughout the marriage, so I'm moving on." I was in this meeting because my husband had stopped coming all together but asked me to continue to come until our official opening because the negativity would have discouraged him from moving forward, and he wanted the appearance of faithfulness to the end. He, instead, went to other churches to be encouraged.

After we started Sunday morning church, we would try to go to their Sunday night service only to feel shade from people we served with and considered to be family for the past decade. I mean people who were the Godparents of our children and we were the Godparents of theirs. It is shameful that the church culture made it so that when you leave a church, you are the enemy and are ostracized. Sometimes family did not speak to each other if their family member left the church. I hate to say it, but it seems a bit cultish to me. God's people have to do better where that is concerned. We are all still a part of God's body, even when we don't serve in the same church.

All that said, we never dealt with the things that happened to us, we never went to counseling, we just dived into ministry headfirst, and we never looked back. At least that's what I thought.

Chapter 7
PASTORING

So here we are, officially pastoring the Ananeo Christian Center. Because my husband studied the Greek language, he named the church a Greek word "ananeo" meaning the new and the fresh.

He wanted the experience of our services to feel new and fresh, and he wanted our church to be a place of new beginnings. It was significant to our experience because we were starting over. He also wanted it to be a place of new beginnings for those like us who needed a fresh start. He didn't want the church to look like where we had come from. He even said if I ever become a tyrant, controlling, or made the church so taxing that people could not enjoy their families to always remind him that he didn't want to be that. We decided to only have one service on Sunday morning and one bible study during the week. We wanted people to enjoy their family time after church and to build a life outside of the church. It was great seeing him in this element and not as the young judgmental "dude" I met years ago.

The place was beginning to pack out. By the time we got to spring, people were standing outside the door of our 60-seater space. I had invited people from my job, which was nearby, and they kept multiplying. The members there did the same. But, the place was also beginning to fall apart because it was an old building. One day we came in, and a part of the ceiling had collapsed. The pews almost couldn't hold the people. They were old wooden pews, and the paint was chipping on all of them. My husband had gotten a call (I'm assuming) from a pastor that he preached for saying that she was closing down her church, and she wanted to know if he could use any of her furniture. That was a blessing from the Lord because we pulled those pews out and replaced them with her chairs. Some of her members even came to join our church, including an awesome young man who, to this day, is a phenomenal musician and sought out drummer, which was a blessing to our ministry.

During this year, my husband's grandmother passed away. Now, this was the woman who raised him, and throughout him planning and taking care of the entire funeral, I noticed that I hadn't seen him cry at all. When I mentioned this to him, he told me to stop looking for him to cry because he was okay. I was confused, because in my mind, if this was the woman that raised you and was so dear to you and also a pillar in your life, there should be some emotion shown during this time or at her funeral. He did mention that he wished that he was there for her a little more at the end, but other than that, I didn't see him show any emotion.

Also, within a short timeframe, his first pastor, who started the church he grew up in, passed away. This also affected him deeply, as he did mention that, but still, there was no great show of emotion as if this was somebody that was so dear to him. At the funeral, was a childhood friend of his who played the organ and sang awesomely. He had recently left his church, and after sitting and talking with him, he and his beautiful wife decided to come over to our church. I remember her being beautiful and pleasant. The first Sunday that they came, you can tell that she was looking around like, "Oh Lord, where are we, and why are we here?"

This childhood friend was a blessing, as he could play and sing. The very first service they attended, my husband had to speak that afternoon. We all went with him to the service. She and I hit it off right away. We laughed at the same things, we talked about having the same experiences, and after church and eating, we had such a great time. This woman became one of my very best friends. When her marriage was ending, and she needed support, we would pick her up, and she would hang at the house for days. This brought us even closer. We enjoyed the same music, and literally, I had been through a bad marriage already, so we connected and shared our most intimate stories. Then she became family when my grandmother, my rock, passed away in 2009, and she spent days with me as I tried to make it through that.

The church was growing out of our small location. We began to search for new buildings. It was April 2006 that we found the location that we believed could hold our ministry.

It was a matter of six weeks, and we had designed, sheetrock, painted, and had a church. This location looked like construction had gone wrong, but after my husband had negotiated with the contractor, we turned it into a wonderful ministry.

The first day that we had our official service in our new location, it had to be over 150 seats in the sanctuary, and it was packed. Everyone was so proud of our accomplishments; they brought their family and friends to this auspicious occasion. People had mentioned that they been in many churches where there was a building fund, and the church never got a building. However, when we did our building fund, we had a church within a couple of months, and it was beautiful. At this point, we were established. I didn't have to do anything anymore. We formed an usher board, trustee board, and an incredible praise team. He was being called out to preach to places all over the city and out of state.

That first year of pastoring, he didn't want to have guest speakers because he wanted his sheep to know his voice. So, I preached when he was out, and that was always scary for me coming behind such a remarkable preacher. Although he taught us how to preach, I always felt I could not live up to him. I was also being called the "first lady" now, too, in which I had people trying to tell me what that looked like, including my husband. You have to walk a certain way; you have to talk a certain way. I even had people telling me what I was supposed to wear! It was always the same: long dresses, hats, and stockings that irritated my legs! By the end of each service, the hat was off because I was a passionate praiser, and I was hot, and the hat felt confining. I would rip my stockings off before the benediction.

After a lengthy amount of time trying to fit the mold, I had a heart to heart with God. God let me know that it was okay to be myself. By being transparent and unapologetically myself, I found that I saw a difference in the response of the people when I ministered. I stopped wearing hats and stockings! But I was authentic, warm, and welcoming. People can tell when you are not being yourself, and it's uncomfortable for everyone. I was decent for church; no body parts hanging out, but fashionable and being the fashionista I always loved being since a child. I could be wrong, but people appreciated and loved the real me. I prided myself in being a down to earth, touchable, cool, first lady.

After a year, we began to have conferences and have guest speakers. He was a great strategizer; he started to call in the great names of the city to put our church's name on the map.

Every great name he brought in, he would prophesy accurately, and they formed relationships after. This strategy was working. We began to become the talk of the city. People were asking, "Who's that young man over there having good church?" The band began to flow, and I even wrote a welcome song for our church. Some awesome singers started to draw to our church, making it an incredible sound. We were becoming known as the one-two punch: great praise and worship and a great word. We started growing rapidly at that location as well; so much so, that he decided that we needed to go to pastors and leader church conference in Texas to be able to handle such church growth in excellence.

The conference was terrific. The leaders had five churches, and they all had thousands of members. We saw pastors there that we knew, and the information that we received was priceless. Every time we came back from conferences like this, we were on fire and ready to do ministry on another level. I would take the information from these conferences and gather a team of administrators and excellent workers to make manuals for every intricate part of our church.

To this day, I believe I could take those manuals and help people start their churches. It was such useful information, and we took it and made it our own, fit for our church. I tried to get him in on making the manuals, but he insisted that I knew what he wanted, and I just needed to make it happen.

The only thing about coming from these conferences is that I think it made my husband question himself and what he was doing and believing. We were a foot-stomping, old school, shouting and speaking in tongues, radical church. It was what people came to our church to experience. The pastor at the church in Texas testified once that after being Pentecostal for some time, the Lord told him to sit the people down and teach them. He said he had 300 members, and 270 of them left because they wanted the Pentecostal move. However, that pastor said he didn't regret it, and sitting the congregants down and becoming a teacher was the best thing that happened to his ministry; hence he has several mega ministries including, all of the pastors that are, under his leadership across the country.

After coming back from the conference, my husband said he was going to sit the people down and teach them. I believe he desired to have a mega ministry. He began to mock our emotional services. We were pretty much nondenominational because he grew up Baptist, and his prophetic was groomed in a Pentecostal church. He also said the day that he got saved was at an Apostolic church that his godmother used to take him to after his morning services. So, I always used to joke that we were "apostolibapticostal" because we were a little bit of all of that. I will say everything I learned about ministry, preaching, protocols, the different sects of ministry was from my husband. He grew up in church, and he observed everything and incorporated it into our church. But now he wanted to put an end to all of the emotionalism.

After service, he always asked me how I thought it went. I'm not going to lie- the teaching was incredible. I always loved good teaching, principles that you can take home and do your best to live out. However, a praising church was ultimately how our church had grown, and I honestly didn't see anything wrong with praising God. You have the radical people that would praise God a lot, and those that would just clap their hands and worship God in their own way. I didn't think you had to knock one to do the other. Some told him that they enjoyed this teaching delivery more. But then some needed that emotional praise, but he somehow made them feel bad about it.

After some time, he couldn't help himself. He would take off the lapel mic and get right back to good old school preaching and praising God. Sometimes he couldn't even get to a sermon, and we wound up praying and worshiping in the service. I expressed that he should be himself and let the Holy Spirit guide him. Ultimately, I love good praise and loved excellent teaching. He did both well. So, I suggested that he start out teaching the sermon and that we end in celebratory praise. This might just be me, but it was the best of both worlds, and all needs would be met. As a wife, I watched him many years down the line fight with who he was and who he wanted to portray. I never forget when he found out that a pastor didn't want to have him at their church because he was too radical. I remember him bashing that pastor and saying that they were just jealous. I believe everyone has a preference, and you won't always be everyone's choice, but you will be chosen to go where you are preferred!

He started the ministerial board, as he had done at our old church, and begin to teach us how to preach and the protocol of ministry. This was awesome because whenever he had to preach during out during the days, we had service, I had to take over the service and preach. I was always so afraid to preach because he was so awesome, I thought that the people would not receive me. But somehow, just like singing, once I grabbed the mic, it always worked. He was very critical of preachers and singing, so that never really helped with my insecurities or my fear of standing before the people. He always told us he criticizes us to make sure that we are the best at what we do. We always took that as love; however, it made us very fearful of going forth. It also didn't help that if he didn't like something, he couldn't hold his face.

With the church multiplying, he was finally able to go to the accountant and was told he could receive a salary and housing from the church. That, along with his many speaking engagements, positioned us to be able to afford to build a house from the ground up. We moved far out on Long Island to get a bang for our buck. It was an hour to get to and from our church. Before we moved there, he traded in my car that I paid off for an Escalade. It was needed because when we picked up the kids, our car was packed. Things were looking amazing for us.

Our church was growing and doing well, we began to form relationships with some of the greats of the city, and I loved everything about worshiping and serving at my church. I started an addiction recovery group, which brought in some great members. I would always try to find stuff that we can do outside of the preaching services. Group ministry has always been my heart. I always felt like preaching to people is good, but we could get to know each other better one on one, and people can get a lot of questions answered. I also started a new members' class, where I would teach the new members about our church and salvation. Looking back now, the intimate settings was something that he left to us all the time. I even started some marriage ministry groups and tried to have a women's fellowship. When people would come with proposals about outreach, he would always tell us that we didn't have what we needed to get those things started. To this day, I don't understand why he didn't push outreach ministry. I missed outreach like prison ministry, nursing homes, and going to shelters.

Before we moved into our home, my husband convinced me that we needed to have a child together. And with his convincing, I agreed. He said if our other children decided to go and be with their other parents, we needed one that would be ours to take care of us. After agreeing, I stopped using my IUD and became pregnant immediately. That was short-lived because, during the sonogram appointment, we realized there was no heartbeat. I remember standing up before the people doing praise and worship as I've done every single Sunday but not being able to make it through that without breaking down and crying. I didn't realize that that miscarriage had affected me so much until then. I didn't think about it much, but when we moved into our house, a month later I found out that I was pregnant again. Any woman that has been through a miscarriage knows those doctor visits are very scary not knowing if this baby will be alive. Well, at this point, my baby was alive. Soon, we had our first son together.

I was traveling back and forth an hour to work while doing ministry faithfully with my husband. By the end of my pregnancy when I couldn't stay up on the road anymore, I took a four-year leave from the New York City Department of Education. Shortly after my son was born, my husband's son's mother had fallen on hard times, and he told me that the boys were going to move in with us as well. We had the big house, and he always said he felt guilty for not having them with him, so this worked out because he wanted his family together. I went from a two-bedroom apartment and one child, stepsons on the weekend to a 3600 square-foot home and four children overnight. It was a tough transition because I still was very involved in my church. At the same time, I was happy that he felt better having them with us.

My husband, on the other hand, didn't do well with children. He could do about five minutes, and then he was done. I would complain about needing help because this was a lot of children, including the newborn. The boys would fight all the time, and we were adjusting to the blended family dynamic, which is a whole other story. I did my best to let the boys see that they were welcome, that we love them, and that they were not my stepsons but my sons. My husband even told them not to call me Janelka anymore but to call me mom. I found myself trying to prove and make them see that I love them like I love my own. Anyone raising a blended family knows it can be challenging.

When my stepsons came, they were very behind in their schooling. They started a new school where only 1% of the students were black children. I didn't want them to go in and be unable to keep up. I remember staying up sometimes to midnight, trying to catch them up to the speed of this new school district. I was a teacher by day, so I did everything I could to get them where they needed to be.

My daughter, on the other hand, had been an A student from kindergarten. From birth till now, she's still the quietest person in the room. She only opens up around close friends and family. This caused a lot of conflict with the oldest. He would often say that she was being favored. He actually was a very smart boy but as time moved on, I realized that he was too smart for his own good. He always got his little brother in trouble and tried to do the least but wanted to receive the most. I would consistently catch him in a lie, and I think he didn't like me because of it. I tried to explain to my kids that I know what you're up to because I was a kid who got into lots of trouble too.

This became hard to balance because you want to be able to reward children for their excellent grades and good behavior, and you have to discipline children for their misbehaving and not doing what they are supposed to do in school. It became a difficult task as the sole disciplinary figure; especially children you didn't give birth to and you're trying to show them that you love them. Therefore, there are times when you don't want to discipline them. I'll never forget being so hurt when my husband's mother came to help me with the children. The eldest had her believing that we were treating him like the black sheep. From two months of her being around, she realized he was trying to play her too, and she wound up cursing him out. Children will play all sides of the fence. Adults have to be on the same page regarding disciplinary actions and stand as a team in order not to be played.

Those are blended family issues. I will say this after, a few years of that I looked my sons in the eye and told them I have shown you nothing but love, as if I gave birth to you myself, there were no favorites, and I will no longer bow as if I have to prove still how much I love you. At some point, I stopped trying to prove my love and just became their mom.

As I mentioned, things were challenging, trying to run the church and raise four children. My husband had his godmother come and help us at times. She was an older woman who cooked well. So, she would help with the meals and babysat when we had to go out to do ministry. At some point, she decided it was too much, and went to go and take care of her home and her husband. Then to make the load lighter, we hired the cleaning company that cleaned the clubhouse to come and clean our house. If I mentioned to my husband about helping around the house, he would say, "I'm paying for a cleaning company." I told him, after I do laundry for a family of six, put away the clothes, clean all 3600 square feet of space so that they can mop, wipe down, and vacuum it was still a lot. He and the kids were messy, and all the while the cleaners did not put things away, they just did the general cleaning, they didn't know where our things belonged. I had done all the work; they just wiped everything down. I still had to do homework with all the children, go to every school event for each child, and even help him carry the weight of ministry. To him, that was nothing. He thought that I had it good.

He told me I had the luxury of being a stay-at-home mom, and that was my sole job, so I should not complain. The funny thing is that during the week he was also home with me. But that was just one of his chauvinistic ways of being a husband and father. Instead of helping, he told me that I could put my two-year-old in daycare. His way of helping all the time was through throwing money at the situation, so he didn't have to do the work himself. I accepted it because I was a stay-at-home mom, and I did start to feel like I should be grateful that I didn't have to work, so my job was to take care of the home and the children. I just made it work. I thought, okay, be a good Christian, please my husband, make sure the kids are fed, clean, educated, getting along and trained, while being a good pastor, first lady, look good myself, and remain balanced. I got this!

Ministry was good to us. One of the things that we learned from the pastoral leadership conferences is to not burn out by going on vacation at least once or twice a year. We went on cruises to many different countries, and we traveled every year during our anniversary week. I was so grateful because I never got to travel like this growing up. He started to buy me beautiful things like Louis Vuitton and Louboutin shoes, which became my signature shoe. I always loved shoes from a little girl. So, this made me very happy. We knew the "Who's Who" in ministry and became a part of the "Who's Who" in ministry. He prided himself on buying me the best of everything, which I know now by the way he bragged about it made him look good too.

The only people that he would hang out with was a handful that had been with us from the beginning. He made a few of them trustees because they had been with us since the beginning, they believed in his ministry, and were able to be his friends and respect him as their pastor at the same time.

This is awesome, but the only problem with your congregants being your friends, now looking at it from a distance, is how much of it is a friendship when they reverence you as their leader. This can only work if, when needed, you can separate the two. So, whenever we went to restaurants, he sat at the head of the table, told everybody where to sit. When conversations were being had, he would lead the conversation, and if you had a difference of opinion, he continued to draw you into his persuasion. As I talk about it with this particular group of people today, talking about relationships always made all the other couples go home arguing. Sometimes I would zone out of the conversations, partially because I didn't always agree and because I was tired of hearing him lead and direct every conversation.

I would go home and tell him that he needed to be careful about calling out a man in front of his wife. He did well talking to women and counseling women, especially older women. But when you are talking to your friends, I explained that they have a right to run their homes the way they want and that he could always learn from a difference of opinion. He was always the alpha male at the table, but most men let it ride because they humbly reverenced the title. He explained because he grew up and learned from women that he knew how to deal and counsel them better.

Either way, we adjusted to this lifestyle. He wanted to have another child because he said he always wanted his daughter, and he wanted to see if he could make a girl. I totally disagreed. He kept trying to convince me that he would pay for all the things I needed to help me. I didn't care. I would be the one who would have to give up my body; wake up at night, and adding a 5th child to our family would be a lot. So, we continued to do ministry. Every time we came back from a conference, we had better ideas. At this point, we hired a day staff at the church. I couldn't work at the church, but I made sure my meeting was after or before service time. I made sure all the kids did what they had to do in school; everyone had clean clothes, including all of my husband's needs were met. Many titles were added to my ministry. As the Pastor of Worship and Arts, I had meetings and rehearsals weekly, and I was managing the dance department and drama department when we had theatrical plays. We always tried to get a helper from the church to come and put a little money in their pocket. However, I wanted everything done a certain way, so I was hands-on when they did. The one thing that kept me anxious and confused was we never had a set schedule.

There is a saying in the church world that prophets are moody. I used to agree-- living with a prophet seeing that he would change moods and ideas week after week and month after month. However, with my lifelong education in psychology, I now understand moody is a personality trait. When it affects your family, relationships, work ethic (etc.) negatively for long periods, it could be a mental disorder.

We started out having a Sunday morning service at 11 AM, then there we changed the service times to 12 PM. He suddenly felt that we were so packed out that we needed a 10 AM and a 12 PM service. Then, the Lord said to start a church in Brooklyn. At this point, we had a 9 AM in Brooklyn and the 12 o'clock in Queens. That was a little daunting because the same people who ministered and helped in Brooklyn had to now rush over to minister and help in Queens. We still were not doing community outreach; therefore, we would just overuse the same people at both churches.

Out of nowhere, he said the Lord told him to shut down the church in Brooklyn. I remember some competent ministers could have been able to keep our church in Brooklyn going, and with their autonomy, who knows what success they could have had at that location. We were renting the building from another pastor, and to back up what my husband had said the Lord said, he complained that they weren't keeping the building tidy and the fact that they were renting out their multi-usage space to people having parties, that there was a spirit in the church. I now know that a lot of what the Lord said were the things that he said to back up the changes he wanted to make.

Another example is when he said the Lord told him to change the name of the church. No one could understand the word Ananneo, and we always had to explain what it meant. People even passed by and read the sign and thought it wasn't an English-speaking church. There didn't have to be a "thus saith the Lord" on that decision, as changing the name so that people could understand it was a legit reason. It made marketing and advertisement a lot easier.

People do not like to admit this, but leading and running a church is like running a business if you want it to grow healthy and run successfully. Making good marketing decisions, investments, and treating the people with excellent customer service can be useful to the growth (and that's not just in numbers) of the ministry. Growth can mean that the people are growing, their lives are being transformed, investments are being made, and the church is maintaining. So, then we only had service in Queens again. That was fine with me because two churches and all of those services were too much for me.

I have always believed in the leading of the Lord. I think that the Holy Spirit has been protecting, leading, and guiding me even before I accepted Christ as my Savior. However, as a Christian, we have to delineate between our common sense, education, and our voice that just wants what we want. Holy Spirit is a gentleman, and at the end of the day, we have choice power. There were times that we raised building funds to change the church around to fit the people and the growing needs of the church. But then there were times that schedules were moved for no apparent reason other than that he just didn't have the capacity to stick with it anymore. Then other times, when he was on what I call 1000, he wanted to clean out and throw out everything and would call everyone to drop what they were doing because he wanted it done by yesterday. This is what I had to endure eventually at church and home with a family of seven.

I remember when the boys' mom moved down South, she got settled and wanted the boys back. I was so hurt, and I worked so hard to get them where they were in school, I didn't want them to go. But I understood that that was their mother and she has a right to raise them. The only problem is it was only about three more weeks left before one of the boys graduated from elementary school, and he said that she wanted them right away. To this day, I cannot understand why they could not agree to allow him to go to graduation before they left. I almost wonder now, being that I never had conversations with their mother, if this was even something that she would not bend on. I learned that a lot of what he was doing always had some other motive and didn't always add up.

Once the boys were there, they started complaining after while about not liking their mother's husband. So, he decided he was going to rescue his boys and bring them back home. I then had to go up to the school and explain to them why they had to come back in the middle of the school year. He never went to these meetings with me because he didn't want to have to face the same embarrassment that I had to face in getting them back to school. But I did it. I was happy to have them again- I had missed my family. But then, the oldest didn't like the rules that were made here, and he began to get upset and decided he wanted to go back down South with his mom.

I told him just because you don't get what you want here; you don't get to jump up and move. His father had a conversation with his mother, and they decided to let him go, and his little brother followed. My husband and I argued about this because children should not get to choose and decide when they don't want to obey rules and move. But the agreement was that if he goes, he does not come back. He had to finish out his schooling down South.

After the boys had moved down South, they again were having a tough time dealing with their mother's husband. I'll never forget having this conversation in front of one of the brothers in the church that was his driver at the time. He said the boys are coming back, they are not getting along with their mother's husband, and I'm their father, and they're getting older, they shouldn't have to deal with another man. I told him that we needed to put our foot down as parents, and we told them if they left again, they couldn't come back. I knew as an educator; you cannot keep flipping back and forth with the emotions of children. They will not learn, and they will think that they can do and get whatever they want when they want.

Well, he put his foot down; and I think it was because he was trying to be a macho man in front of that brother, but told me, "I spoke to their mother, this is my house, and those are my sons, and I said they're coming back to move with me." I remember being very embarrassed and hurt. He always had conversations with their mother, and decisions were made without my consent even though when they were with us, I was the one raising them. I can say I resented him for that conversation for many years. I did all the hard work, but I never had a say so. And guess who went to the school in the middle of the school year to get them back in school? Imagine trying to explain why they had to keep going back and forth. His choices in those scenarios showed a lot of his mood swings in making decisions.

Anyone who knows me and worked ministry with me can attest to this. We always chalked it up to him being a visionary on the move. But I began to question the instability.

He would argue with me that I wasn't the pastor, and God speaks to him about what this church has to do. He would say things like, "If it's broken, throw it out. If it's not working, fix it." My only issue with that was he never let things play out long enough to see if it would work. I learned from my women's meetings that as long as I'm consistent, some things will grow, it started with just a handful of women. But as I continued to have the meetings every month, it began to grow and multiply. I began to do something called the Harvest Café because now we were Harvest Church International. This is where people would come with their talents to sing, dance, poetry, and play instruments. It started very small, but over time we were packing out the church. Consistency is key to growth!

I hate to say it, but as much as he tried to convince us that he moved in an excellent spirit, consistency was something he lacked. The only problem was he was the master at making you believe what he wanted you to think about him, which I know now he didn't believe himself. Some of the things that I see about him now, I didn't know while I was in it. The bad part was if anyone mentioned or confronted his inconsistencies, he would then isolate them, remove them, or make sure everyone around them believed the negative things he said about them. He had a way of adding in their faults and flaws to make sure all that he spoke to accepted and believed in the negativity.

My studies on narcissists show that they do this to make sure since those people see them for who they are, if they expose it, they will not influence the people they have tainted. Those people eventually left the ministry. They were always in the wrong, not him. I didn't still know this was happening. I believed they all were haters, jealous, and just against him because he was favored.

Well, we will now see with those who worked outside of us, like when we joined a large organization, how it revealed who he was or what was happening around us. He was the leader at our church, but when you join an organization with your peers, you can't influence them like the people under you. They don't have to do what you say, and you can't manipulate other prophets with your gift. He thought he could, but he found out quickly.

Chapter 8

I KNEW SOMETHING WAS WRONG: MENTAL ILLNESS REVEALED

In my husband's questioning being a good leader, he talked about getting his divinity/theology degree. I thought that would be great because I know I always wanted to go back to school for my master's degree, but after getting married and having babies, the family became the priority. However, we did have people that were helping us in the home and the church was doing so well that as we discussed going back to school, we talked about going back to school together. There was a Christian school called Nyack College that had a theology degree and also had a master's in clinical counseling. This was awesome because I had been counseling members in our church without a degree in this area, and I felt that it would be nice to have the education to back it up. He had been preaching for many years and had taken several Old and New Testament classes. This would complete his education.

I had to take some prerequisite courses before the semester started online. After getting my children to bed, I would stay up late at night to complete my coursework. I ended up getting two A's, and I was so proud of myself. He would always tell me that I was smart but that he was smarter than me, and if I needed help with my schoolwork, he would help me. I always took those as joking moments. However, when we began to start the semester together, he started to get stressed out. What I didn't know then is that he had a bit of anxiety when it was time to do papers. He always bragged about getting into the classroom and answering all the questions, and his classroom participation was excellent. He did not have a bachelor's degree, but he was able to talk to different people in the school and was able to get into the master's degree program without a bachelor's degree. To this day, I don't know how he was able to do that, but I chalk that up to his gift of gab. He was that good.

So now he's having a very difficult time completing his papers and when I asked if he wanted my help that became a problem. He started to say things like, "I don't really need this degree" or "I already am doing everything that I want to do in ministry, so why get this degree?" Plus, the ministry needed his attention, and somehow the Holy Ghost was leading him in another direction. I wound up getting A's and B's that semester, and I think his might've been incomplete. By the end of the semester, we didn't have that driver anymore, and I was taking the train to school by myself. I loved it, though. I loved getting my degree.

At the same time, I'm also getting involved in the organization as a singer and praise and worship leader. One of the ministers of music had worked with the best of the best in gospel, and I was honored to work with him in ministry. I talked about my dream of recording music. He told me he had a studio and we could work on that. We talk about recording. I was so elated that he would consider that, and I shared it with my husband. He didn't make a big deal about it, but I do remember the next time we saw this producer, he mentioned doing a hymn album. I just remember thinking that I never heard him talking about making any recording, but as soon as I had an opportunity he is trying to plug himself in. Wow. I left it alone because I didn't want to believe the thoughts I was thinking about my husband at that point.

He then started pressing me to have his daughter again. He begged, saying, "Please let me have this" and talked about how since he was a good father who takes care of his children, one more won't hurt. He was so convincing, but I wondered, "What if it's not a girl?" But the same prophet that came in and prophesied that after I had my miscarriage, I would have full-term baby, who didn't even know I had a miscarriage, prophesied that the next baby if I wanted to, would be a girl. I remembered that prophecy, and I thought if I was going to have another baby, I guess I wouldn't mind having a baby girl. They were smarter, easier, they moved a little faster, so I stopped using birth control.

I didn't get pregnant right away, and the new school semester was getting ready to start. At this time, my husband still was not a lot of help to me, because he became isolated in his world. But I decided to go back to school anyway. Of course, I got pregnant right after. That didn't last very long because without his help, and without transportation, I was getting big fast, and I really couldn't do it all. I told the Dean that I'm going to take a break and come back after I had the baby. She encouraged me to do so, saying that I was a bright student. His mom came from down south to help with the kids. He convinced her that she needed to stay and help. He felt that since she didn't raise him, she needed to come down and see her grandkids growing up. She was single, used to living alone, and didn't want to make this lifestyle change, but she loved her son and moved down on the condition that she had to get her place. Honestly, it was a relief for me, as I needed the help, so I looked tirelessly until I found a place that took her Section 8.

The success of the church made him worse because one of the well-known Bishops (Fathers) in the city, who had a lot of influence on many of the young preachers, welcomed my husband and acknowledged his gifting. He had been asking some of the other guys about my husband and the ministry, and everyone had something good to say.

This Bishop invited him to preach at one of his well-known events in the city. This was a huge opportunity for exposure because some of the greatest pastors and ministers from across the country have been a part of this event. The invitation made my husband feel amazing, and he was so proud to share the news with everyone. However, a few days prior to the event, that Bishop called him and said there had been a change and that he was not going to be able to speak at the event. I remember my husband being extremely hurt, trying to identify what he had done wrong or what could have been said about him that led to him being canceled.

Instead, we got dressed up and went to the event anyway. We were prepared to give our offering and then leave. We arrived at this big movie house theater. It was the most beautiful church, and it was huge! The Bishop spotted us coming in and told the ushers to bring us right to the stage with the other preachers. They had an awesome talk after the service, and the Bishop told my husband that the Lord told him to make him a bishop, but he didn't know how he was going to do it if he wasn't a part of the organization. Well, my husband joined the organization, and he became a bishop. Being under somebody else really exposed my husband's insecurities. He worried about what that man thought about him all the time.

The minute that my husband started preaching in this organization, there wasn't an event where he wasn't on the program. He would go to the meetings and come back with stories of some of the older gentlemen deciding to leave the organization because they were jealous of the younger guys that were doing everything. There was another young preacher who was excellent, and they began to hit it off. We begin to go out of town and preach for them as well. This opened up doors for my husband on another level. He started saying, "I don't really need this title, and I'm just going to do the work of the Lord." There was a prominent bishop who was part of another large organization that criticized the Archbishop in New York about making all these young guys bishops. I could tell that bothered my husband because that was a massive organization of bishops that a lot of the "Who's Who" fellowship in that he could've possibly been a part of, but he never did.

The Day I Committed Suicide

Shortly after becoming a bishop, my husband started withdrawing from almost everyone. I remember our friends remarking about how he had started "acting funny" since he was ordained as a Bishop, but what they didn't realize is that he wasn't acting funny; he had completely isolated himself from everyone. Some of our closest friends found it severe enough to come over and do an intervention, which led to him exposing their flaws and what was wrong with them, and him saying there was nothing wrong with him. However, at that point, they knew something wasn't right.

Studies reveal that the effects of perceived social isolation across the life span can wreak havoc on an individual's physical, mental, and cognitive health. I am sharing this, mainly because, as Christians and people of color, we need to take aggressive action when we see these symptoms in our loved ones. From my experience, it just continues to get worse over time, and the affected individual's crisis can negatively impact their family, friends, co-workers, parishioners, and others!

For me, I noticed that my husband was very conflicted with the title of "bishop." So, on the one hand, he is saying that he never asked to be a Bishop (almost like it didn't matter to him), but on the other hand, I know that it did because he was so well-versed in everything that went along with the office. I mean, he knew all the regalia, all of the garb, the garments, what the colors meant and everything. He bragged about his lineage of the Bishopric that could be traced back to the Catholic Church, so clearly, all of this was a big deal. I believe though that while it was an honor for him, it was also so big that it scared him.

I am convinced that the weight of the call and the office is one of the chief factors that led to his isolation. In truth, the ministry can create lonely periods for the men and women of God that accept the call. In the bible, there were times where Moses, Joseph, Jeremiah, and even Jesus were all alone in the enormity of the call and the plan of God for their lives. The difference is that in modern times, there are so many other factors of ministry that exist. For example, after my husband was inducted at this level of ministry with all of these other successful clergy that he had to interact with what I will call the "Boys' Club" for lack of a better term, he faced a somewhat healthy competition. Even though it is not really revealed among the laypeople, these guys sit around and discuss how well so-and-so can preach, how many people a particular church has, who is anointed and who is not, and conversations like that.

I believe that's what caused the later demise in his mental facilities. Events with other men in high positions, coupled with the pressure of being a bishop, just created significant duress. Also, trying to live up to the "image" and "expectation" of others while trying to manage your church well, with the added pressure of planting other churches (for which he didn't have a plan). There was another young bishop that became a bishop with him from out of town, and he already had a handful of churches under his belt. I told him to get with him and figure out how he's doing what he's doing.

Another factor I remember taking a toll on him was the many attempts to get a new building for this growing church—one time, we put down $50,000 on an auction building that didn't come through. We were referred to another pastor with a large building but not many members. After thinking that he was getting close enough to receive favor, this pastor started asking for $3 million—something we absolutely could not afford. There was another older pastor with a large church not too far from us, that when he passed away, the children took over even though he said he would consider him. There was a lot across the street from the church in which he spoke to the owner, and the owner said maybe in a couple of years we could purchase it, but when he died, their children sold it, and they made a bunch of stores. The last attempt was a man who owned a lot of buildings in our town. His daughter happened to be a member of our church. But he began to get old and senile, and trying to speak with him to work out a deal for one of his locations was like trying to find a needle in a haystack.

I was there for most of the negotiations. I was there every night that he talked about what he would do with the buildings when he thought we were going to get them. I was also there to see the look in his eyes of disappointment whenever these buildings didn't come through. It was like his gift of gab wasn't working anymore, or the favor that was on the ministry seem to be fading. We prayed and shouted every week for our new building. More people, larger buildings, and constant progress would signify success. But it didn't seem like that was happening anymore.

So, we moved on to the next thing. The plan was to get the church moving with the times of technology and social media. The truth is, we always had state of the art equipment. If we were going to have something, he always wanted it to be the best of the best. We stayed in the music stores. He stayed online, researching the best of the best. Even in our home, we always had to have gadgets that made things easier. I called my husband a "gadget whore," and in turn, he called me a "shoe whore." We had big TV screens on the wall, so whenever we did a building fund, we always bought some more state-of-the-art equipment. We prided ourselves on being a well-kept, state-of-the-art church that use funds to beautify the church.

Around this time, I was starting to get the church online and increase our presence digitally. I was helping to cast vision to the team as it related to what he wanted to do next, which involved getting iPads, new church software to offer text messages for offerings and to communicate and manage our church membership. Next, we would be purchasing screens and have additional software to enable us to do check-ins for Children's Ministry. I was giving direction to each team and training them on what they needed to do. For example, the church membership software allowed us to e-blast our members via email.

It was a truly remarkable system, and I would stay up sometimes until 3 a.m. learning the features and components of the software. We would continuously meet about making the church better and new. It was around this time that I started to notice a more severe change in my husband. It seemed that by the time I would learn new software, he was trying to replace it and purchase the latest and next best thing, although the one that we had was fine for our needs. I was continually trying to get him to make a choice so that we could move forward.

The Day I Committed Suicide

Shortly after this, one day, I was with a college student from our church who served as a mommy-helper. She was telling me how she struggled to write a paper until her friends gave her Adderall. She said this helped her to stay up and write an entire paper in one night.

After this, my husband went to our family doctor and told her that he had ADHD, and she prescribed him Adderall. Now, it is possible that he did have it because our younger two children were diagnosed with it; however, they took a test to determine their diagnosis, and he didn't... he just gave her symptoms. Over time, I would watch him read about symptoms, and he would then diagnose himself. Then he would tell our family doctor of these symptoms to get the meds he wanted.

When I spoke to one of his close friends after everything had been revealed, he said, "Yeah, your husband was always a hypochondriac." Every time that I got sick, which was not very often, he would immediately say, "I must have the same thing" and lay down in the bed with me. I used to get angry because I felt that he only got sick with me so that he wouldn't have to take on my responsibilities. I could never be sick alone. We also laughed about that, and I don't know if that was just him being lazy or hypochondria.

This is where things began to get noticeably worse. First, we had a pastor friend who was only 40 to have a stroke, and he almost died. This sent him spiraling. I noticed a change in his preaching. He would take the Adderall just before preaching, and his introduction would be super-long and all over the place, sometimes never getting to his points. This was noticeable for me because he taught us how to preach and criticized anyone who would preach the way he was starting to preach. Then, he declared a total lifestyle change. The problem was every month he changed it. No exaggeration. One month he was pescatarian, then he said a piece of fish got him very sick, and so the next month, he becomes a vegetarian, and he was juicing. It seemed like every week or every month; my husband discovered a new trend or diet.

Now, after my formal training, I see that all of this was manic behavior because it didn't stop there. He started buying all of this equipment to work out. After one day of working out with a friend who was a personal trainer, he said he couldn't breathe, and he never went back to working out. Next thing you know, he has all these pumps, and he said that he had exercise-related asthma. We all just believed him, but again, when I look back now, he diagnosed himself with a lot of things and wasn't even going to the doctor. He did have our family doctor who he would give a whole bunch of symptoms and was able to come back with the medications that he wanted. Half of the things that he said was wrong with him now I don't even know if it was true.

I now believe he was acting as the result of a fear of death that started when our pastor friend had that stroke but was made worse by a cousin of his who suddenly died from an asthma attack, and he had to do her funeral. On top of that, the cousin's dad died two weeks later. I watched his personality completely change because he was not dealing with the impact of their deaths. He was not allowing himself to grieve. In both situations, his family expected him to be the pastor that provided comfort and also provided financially for some of the expenses of these funerals. It was a tough time for him, and he kept getting worse. His preaching style continued to shift and increase in length. He was long-winded, seemed scattered, and seemed to have no concept of time when he was on the podium.

The Adderall that had been prescribed by our family doctor added to the intensity of the situation. He began taking it more and more, and he would stay up all night, read several books, do a little project around the house, and be convinced that the pills were helping him. He listened to all kinds of audiobooks, saying he could finally get through books. He was an audible learner, and the Adderall was helping him to get through everything. I also noticed him regularly drinking Red Bull or Five Hour Energy drinks. I was ignorant about this, but I learned that he was finding ways to have the doctor increase his dosage or find a mix of stimulants to give him. I now know that this was a complete overdose of stimulants.

Later, he had two aunts pass away in a close timeframe, and this "death phobia" just completely engulfed him. He was convinced he was dying. He bought multiple machines to check his pulse, and he was checking it all the time. I kept all of this to myself and continued to pray for my husband. Then one day, he lost it. We were at a gas station driving back from the South after one of his aunts died and he jumps out of the car and tells me that his heart is stopping. I told him that I was sure it wasn't, because he would drop dead if it was, but if it was, we needed to head to the hospital. Before I could finish my sentence, he ran into the gas station and bought caffeine pills and took them.

I was starting to panic because his eyes were bulging, and he was talking fast while trying to explain to me that his heartbeat would speed back up when he walked and prayed. All the while, I knew that even with my limited knowledge of the body, that caffeine pills would certainly raise his heart rate. By then, I knew we had to go to the hospital. When we got to the hospital, he kept obsessing with the monitors, and every time he felt that his heart rate was going down, he would jump off the table.

The doctor was obviously looking at him as if this was absurd. Then the doctor asked him what type of medication he was on. He then informed him of the Adderall and Vyvanse, along with the caffeine pills that he had ingested at the gas station. The doctor told him that it was the equivalent of taking speed, which explained his behavior. The doctor's response upset him, and he started bashing the doctor, telling him that he knows that he doesn't recognize his condition as an actual illness, but that he has ADHD and he needs his Adderall. That was the first time I saw him try to protect and defend this drug as if his life depended on it.

The doctor called me out of the room and asked me if my husband has a mental illness. I assured the doctor that he didn't. The doctor was not convinced and told me that my husband had a fixation regarding his heart-stopping, which I did not disagree with, but I was not ready to admit that he may have a mental illness. When I came back into the room, my husband instantly asked me what the doctor said to me. I told him that I told the doctor that he did not have a mental illness, and at that point, my husband decided that the doctors could not help him, and we left and went to a hotel room.

However, I did tell my husband that I thought that the doctor was not wrong about the symptoms, and maybe we needed to change his prescription.

That one statement sent him over the top and made me the enemy who sides with all of his enemies. We decided to stay overnight at the hotel, and he agreed that I could not stay in his room because I was the enemy. After being in my room for less than an hour, I hear a commotion in the hallway. I came out of my room to my husband yelling and screaming with a towel around his waist in the hallway. The cops were called, and he was taken out of the building. His mother, aunt, and I were screaming and crying. They put him in an ambulance, and we were heading back to the hospital. He seemed to think that the doctor must've called the hotel and told them that he was crazy. They wound up giving him some Benadryl to calm him down, and he chalked it up to him just having an allergic reaction to something at his aunt's house. Several of our friends and ministers drove all the way down to make sure he was okay. I watched him tweak the entire event for sympathy and justification. All of the running in the streets, yelling, taking caffeine pills, mixed with two other stimulants that he was taking, being taking out by cops, all sounded like a story of injustice and not the circus it was. This was clearly a panic attack that I hadn't put together then. This was the beginning of many incidents that I stayed quiet about that he normalized.

Now he is picking arguments with me, and I am just trying to cling to my sanity. At the same time, my husband continued to use Adderall, and his behavior became more extreme and uncontrollable. This wasn't the first time I heard this next statement, but it was stated more often now. He said I didn't love him like I loved my last husband, and this is why I am not concerned about his well-being. I would often explain, "First of all I was a kid when I married him; second of all, you don't know how I showed him love and that the relationship was short-lived; third, I didn't know anything about love then; and finally, I've been with you triple the years I was with him, and I can't believe that he is still a conversation." I then started accusing him of not getting over that entire situation, which he hated to hear, but it was the truth if he was still talking about it over a decade later.

There were a few panic attacks after that and several stomach issues, which caused him to go to the bathroom all the time. I started to do a lot of research and going back to my old books. He was suffering from an anxiety disorder, which also affects the body. It was irritable bowel syndrome (IBS). He yelled at me for saying that he had anxiety, and he even yelled at me for saying he had IBS. Every Wednesday, he would get sick, and I had to preach for him. I hated that because I didn't like to have to preach the last minute. I liked to have prepared messages.

My cousin had started a cleaning business and would come over a couple of days a week to help me. She said every Wednesday after he laid down and cried out that he was so sick, and after I would close the door to head to the church, he would get up and start building something that he had ordered or doing some other projects around the house as if he wasn't even sick at all. She hesitated to tell me, but after a few weeks of this, she did.

The Day I Committed Suicide

People began to slip away and stop coming around us altogether. It was getting weird, and he was getting mean. He started cursing out the office staff, and one day he went to the church and began whipping computers out of the church. For the next two years, he was obsessed that someone was hacking us and trying to take everything that we had. He spent thousands of dollars on spyware to keep "the people" from taking stuff from us. He bought several camera sets to put around the house, which he would also take down thinking that "the people" were spying on us in those cameras. He would snatch phones from our children, saying that "the people" were coming through our phones and our cable boxes. I would tell him that he needed to get out of this funk and needed to see someone to get better. He preached to so many about healing and moving forward, and I believed that it was time for him to get up and move forward. Sometimes I said it in love, but at times I tried to see if tough love would work. He only argued that he didn't want to be the way he was and that he was going to fix all of these problems. Every week he said he was getting closer to fixing it until I had to take over everything in our lives.

In February 2017, every time he finished preaching, he would take a few steps and complain that he couldn't breathe. After we got home, he yelled at me and said he didn't want to keep telling me that he was sick because I have been telling him to get himself together, but he needed to go to the hospital. No matter how many times he said he needed to go to the hospital, I was always the one to go with him. His mother came over and watched the kids, and we went to the hospital. This time he had a pulmonary embolism, which is a deadly blood clot that could go to the heart or lungs and stop his breathing or his heart suddenly. He threw this up in my face, talking about how I made him feel bad about being sick, and when he told me that he was gravely ill, I never wanted to hear him. For the next year, he tried to treat it like it was stage 4 cancer.

The doctors asked him if he traveled for an extended period or sit still for a long time, and he said no. I had to remind him that he sat at the computers for days at a time and laid in his bed, depressed for days at a time when he couldn't "unhack" the computers. While one of the brothers was visiting at the hospital, he yelled at me and told me to get out of the hospital and said that I was blaming his sickness on him. I was so embarrassed that I just cried and left. I had been back and forth into the hospital, bringing him all of his computers, toiletries, and clothes. Every day it was a long list of things he needed at the hospital, and all he ever did was yell at me and tell me that I was a horrible wife after every trip.

The truth is he possibly could've had that embolism from sitting still for long periods, or from the high doses of Adderall mixed with all the other stimulants he was taking. He told everybody he probably had a rare blood disorder, and he began to obsess over taking his blood thinners. His legs were hurting all the time and were inflamed, and he told us that he had some type of autoimmune disease. I honestly don't know if a doctor came up with that idea or not. He became like a paraplegic for the rest of that year. And I was the worst because I didn't know how to take care of him. After so many nights of him keeping me up with the computers, I decided to move downstairs into a bedroom. I needed rest. I had so much on my shoulders. And forget about him looking at me like I was a woman or wife—we hadn't had intercourse for a couple of years at this point.

When I got down to that bedroom, sometimes after taking my kids to school, I got back in the bed and couldn't get out. One time I felt so heavy; I felt like a brick was laying on me. My family let me stay in a room for three days without coming out. I don't think they even noticed. My best friend noticed and asked me why I was always in bed when she called. At first, I would say I don't feel well, but she knew something was not right. But how could anybody know? Everyone just wanted to stay away from this/us based on the feeling they got when they came around.

For the past year, we would bring all his food, clothes, and everything he needed for the bedroom as if he couldn't even walk. But when he wanted to do a project, he was like Superman.

When I started feeling so down and couldn't move (mind you, this only lasted three days and only happened twice), he called his mother and told her that we were leaving him upstairs for dead. He said he had nothing to eat at times and nobody was checking on him. So, I would hear her come in the door, and he would cry out, "Mommy," as if he was a child.

All of a sudden, I was wondering why she was bringing him food and doing his laundry all the time when that was something that I always did. I confronted her about it, and she said, "I'm just trying to help out." I said, "Okay", because I did appreciate the help.

He always took care of paying the bills and all of the paperwork for the house. He told me I might have to start taking over when I noticed that the bills weren't getting paid. I didn't think I could take on another thing. I had gotten our second oldest in college by myself, going back and forth to the school in New Hampshire, I was in the process of getting my daughter into college, there was our other kids activities (gymnastics, dance, orchestra, basketball, because I kept them all busy), the church services, and the day staff (that I took over) that he would not get involved with unless it was to criticize what I was doing. I was already making the money by going to preach at every engagement he was too sick to go to, raising the finances at the church, and then I was being asked to organize and pay the bills. I refused to do it. He always thought someone was hacking us, and getting him to provide money or a card so that I could go shopping or do things for the kids always led to him having an anxiety attack or a panic attack. I struggled to complete the paperwork for our kids' FAFSA because he insisted "the people" were trying to hack us, so much so that I didn't even realize he hadn't filed taxes in two years.

When he started complaining that there were worms in his fingers, I kept saying, "How could that be?" When he showed me, it looked like everyone else's cuticles. I tried to rationalize and even researched if this could be a thing. Also, if he did have a parasite issue, the usual resting place was in the anus. I tried to explain this, but it only added to his belief of me being a horrible and unsympathetic wife. But when he started blaming the invasion of the worms on me, being a nasty, dirty woman, that was it.

I was tired, and one day I said, "I can't do it anymore. I'm not good". I said this to my husband a couple of times. Often times I would walk away when we had arguments, but now he followed me around when I tried to walk away. I just wanted out of it all. I couldn't take it anymore. All the things that he had been saying to me started to get in my head, and I couldn't make it stop. And then there was "That Day"… Him chasing me around calling me dirty, nasty, mean, non-caring, I couldn't get away, so I chose to go away. Chapter 1 explained it all.

Chapter 9
AFTER THAT DAY

After that day, I saw the psychiatrist while in the hospital. She had to evaluate me to make sure that I was okay to go home. After telling her the events that led to me being in this position, she wondered how I survived it all. She told me that this was situational depression, meaning I was placed in a heavy situation that caused me to be depressed. After talking to her about my educational background and clarity about what I needed to do to get strong for my children, she told me I had to get to his doctor and let her know what the Adderall is doing to him and our family. She also said to me that after that, my first steps should be to see a therapist to help me to move forward from here. I did just that.

I left the hospital, and I tried to call his spiritual mother and godmother. His spiritual mother was sad to hear what had transpired, but she knew she couldn't get through to him. His godmother refused to answer my calls for a few days.

When I finally got her on the phone, she told me that nobody said to me that life would be easy and that I just needed to pray. Her harsh response hurt me. I had told her a few years ago that he was using too many pills and taking too many five-hour energy drinks, and it seemed as if she understood. I thought she could get through to him.

But, this is the problem in the church. We had been praying for years for him to get better. I wonder if the congregants realized how many years we'd been praying for him to get better or if they even realized the severity of his condition. When do we move from praying to doing something to help someone get better? Faith without works is dead. I also realize that everyone was praying about a physical sickness and was unaware that there was a mental health issue.

The crew that came to the hospital for me decided to call me weekly (and sometimes daily) to make sure that I was holding up. There were times where after I got off the phone with one, I would call the others back to back just to ensure I was maintaining my mental stability and hearing positive reinforcements to counteract the negativity coming from him.

At this point, he had expressed that he hated me and was getting meaner by the minute. The kids' godfather flew up from the south because their family had moved, and he felt so bad that they moved during such a tough time in our lives. While he was here, we gathered those that were closest to us for intervention. I remember being a little afraid because the last response didn't go well. But things were horrible at this point, and I could use all the help I could get.

When everyone came over, all he did was dismiss everyone arrogantly, telling them about their issues and their problems, telling them they were too late to help him and that he was already on his way to getting better. He made it seem as though I did what I did to embarrass him and that I was the one who had the real problem. He also said that he had been sick for some time and nobody came to see about him, but as soon as I had an issue, everybody came running. It was at that moment that I began seeing the real hate that he had for me, coupled with jealousy. And the truth is, everyone had been trying to be there for him, but he was pushing everyone away. He stopped answering phone calls, and he stopped coming out, and they wanted to tell him that. But again, he didn't want to hear what they had to say. At this point, we all realized that rationalizing with him was impossible. They tried to tell him that the worms in his body were a delusion, but he still wasn't convinced. He was furious at me for inviting them to come to help him. This was when he became vicious, and there wasn't a single day in that house that he didn't brutally curse me out or tell me off.

It really became unbearable after this, but I just tried to make the best of it. It was so bad that at times I started to record him because I didn't think he would believe me if he ever got better. Then there were times when he was so irate that I would press my recorder just in case he tried to hurt us. Right after my incident, I stayed away for couple of days and when I came home our sons (my stepsons 18 and 19 years old) were home. He was yelling and screaming at them to look at the nest in the ceiling. He had opened up the ceiling.

I stayed locked in my room so that I would not have to deal with him. But when I heard him screaming at the boys, I tried to come out to defend them. Being the young men they had become, they told me to stay in the room, as if they were now protecting me from him.

I made an appointment with his doctor (our family doctor) and told her what was going on. All she could say is that every time he complained about the meds not working, she told him to see a therapist. I couldn't understand why she thought it was okay to continue to give him so many psychotropic medications. After I told her everything that transpired, she shared our conversation with him at his next visit, and I thought he was going to kill me. He stormed out of our home, saying he had to get away from me. That evening, he called me on the phone and was calling me all kinds of derogatory names. It was scary, so I hung up. After hanging up on him twice, 2 minutes later, he came in the door like a mad man. If you have never seen a person in the middle of drug withdrawal, you won't understand what I was seeing. He was jittery and pacing. If I didn't have someone at the house, I don't know what he would have done to me. I started to record him while he explained his depression, anxiety, and why he had to convince his doctors to up his doses so many times. The sister that was there was someone that he loved and respected, so he just started pouring it all out. I thought her presence might be a good thing, but he told her how much he hated me and continued talking, saying how he had discussed the doctor into giving him a dose higher than she was supposed to, and he admitted to doubling up on that dosage. It was heartbreaking to watch.

He was a sick man. Our family doctor told him he had to see a psychiatrist to receive these meds now. So, he saw the psychiatrist that my therapist recommended. That was a disaster, because I had to go to the first appointment, and he was so enraged the doctor was afraid for me. The psychiatrist wouldn't give him the dose he wanted and couldn't understand why he was receiving the dose he was getting. After a couple of visits, he made up a story that me, my therapist, and the psychiatrist were conspiring against him. Then he found his way back to the family doctor and was able to get what he wanted. I decided my efforts would only end up making me more of the enemy, so there was nothing I could do. Every gesture made him hate me more and worsened his behavior.

At this point, I could no longer focus on him. Somebody had to remain sane for the well-being of our children. I decided to ignore him and to start working and preparing to take on everything because it didn't seem that he'd be getting better anytime soon. I had no strength to take care of the church anymore, so the other Pastors were going have to hold it down. My family was in need.

It was also at this point that I spent time trying to remove myself from the marriage emotionally. I was already emotionally disengaged from the marriage, but I still continued to see to it that he was well. I could no longer do this if helping him is killing me. He's always been controlling but, I was always able to handle him, and for the most part, fight for my own identity. However, when the mental illness started getting worse, he became really disgusting, emotionally abusive, and mean. He also had been emotionally absent from our marriage for a few years, especially since his focus was always on some insane theory like the computers, worms, and even more crazy theories! So, he wasn't even thinking about our marriage as a love relationship anymore.

It was time out for me trying to make sure that he got better. Time out for me trying to prove that I cared about him, and trying to do everything I knew how to take care of him. At the time, I was trying to convince myself because there was a lot of talk from him, especially after his pulmonary embolism that I wasn't a supportive wife, and I wasn't taking care of him. He never wanted me to hear the doctors' reports, so he stopped telling me about his appointments. I would only find out that he was going to an appointment when his mom walked in the door.

With all that was happening, there was no self-care for me. I didn't even realize that I hadn't been going to the doctor or the dentist. I had been having migraines and was not even realizing that my blood pressure was becoming so high. It was time to take care of me and to rebuild. It was time for me to do what's best for my children and me. One day he was yelling, saying he couldn't afford to give me money anymore and that he was tired of taking care of us. I told him before if we needed money; I never had a problem with going out and getting a job. I have a bachelor's degree, and I was a teacher's assistant before taking leave, and I have many skills under my belt. But every time I mentioned working, he was insulted. Me being a stay at home, mom was a chip on his shoulder and made him feel like a big boss. But I now know that it was also his way of controlling me. Well, I went to my kid's school and applied for a position as a teacher's aide. They didn't have teacher's assistants, so I settled for an aide position.

It was an entry-level position, and I felt awkward because I had run an entire church, was a public speaker and singer and felt like I had way more experience than what I was about to do. Nonetheless, I could pay the credit card bills, my parents' insurance, and continue to buy the kids' clothes that I already had been paying through the allowance that he gave me. I could try to keep that up. I had to let some credit cards go down. It was just a part-time position working 5 hours a day, for $12hr, getting paid every two weeks. The staff at my kids' school loved me, the kids loved me, and my kids love me being in their school, so I stayed. That was in October 2017.

Every single day he would tell us to come upstairs to see the worms that eventually turned into spiders coming out of his ears, nose, and head. This was the new normal. He made holes and scars everywhere; additionally, he scratched his cornea and blamed it on the spiders. His mom would come by, but she told him she wasn't going to look. Sometimes I would go and look because I thought that maybe I was the problem, and he does have a rare disease. Sometimes I didn't want to believe that he was losing it. But what I could not do was lie and tell him I saw something I didn't see. And there were times that I saw the fear, pain, and the need for others to see what he saw in his face. However, I didn't think telling him it was real would be helpful. I wanted him to snap out of it and get better. Unfortunately, mental illness doesn't work like that.

More and more, I just tried to turn off all of my emotions because I could not let this thing affect me again to the point that I didn't want to live anymore. There were times that I wanted to run away because he was still yelling at me and saying that I wasn't supporting him, that I wasn't a good wife, and that I had people thinking he was crazy. At the same time, he also wasn't showing up to his board meetings for the organization. They kept asking me what was going on, and I just kept saying he's still sick. I told everyone who had questions to check on him on their own. Telling people never helped me, and if he ever got better, I didn't want them to see him like that. His livelihood depended on his reputation, and unfortunately, if he got better, they may not forget this time in his life.

This is why I didn't speak out all those years. When you are married to a man of influence, talking about his abuse, addiction, and mental illness can lead to the family losing their livelihood. Leaving means we have to start over alone (which is scary), and as pastors, exposing their weaknesses can discourage the congregants or cause them to lose their faith, which is no good because their faith should be in God and not in man. But covering the man of God was the culture. And yes, to some extent, you should cover your spouse and keep the family business in the home, but not to the point that it's killing you or them. So, without telling the congregation, I stopped going to church altogether. I told the teams that I was in charge of that my kids had games every Sunday, which for the most part, they did. But before things got to this point, I would come to church immediately following their games.

I received an email from NYU (where my daughter

attended), and it had information about getting a master's degree in school counseling online. So, I decided to apply. Wouldn't that be great? My daughter was already there, and if I was going to go back to work, I wanted to do something great and make good money doing it. I already had education experience, counseling credits, and counseling experience. I needed to secure a future for our family, and school counseling would allow me to have summers and weekends off with the kids.

I wrote a kick-ass essay, got references from a principal that I worked with, one of our pastors that was a principal at our church, and the dean of the program I was enrolled at Nyack. She had always asked when I was coming back to finish up. When the acceptance letter came, I cried like a baby. My kids said, "Mommy, why are you crying?" I told them that I didn't think I could pull it off after being a stay at home mom for ten years, being out of school for seven years and starting again at 40. I showed them that we can do and accomplish anything we put our minds to achieve.

A couple of months later, I realized that it was an $80,000 degree and that even with loans, I would owe $3000 every quarter. It was a perfect situation as far as the school coursework because it was in New York, and I only had to go to school for one intensive class. The rest of the classes met online face to face once a week, and I would finish in 2 years. However, we were behind in bills, and I knew that making $12 per hour; it's not going to work.

For some strange reason, my husband wasn't looking at

the logic. He said he was proud of me, that I got in, and we will make it happen. It was shocking to me that he had something positive to say. But I had to make the hard decision that it wasn't going to work. I refused to start and stop because I couldn't pay, and I didn't want to have $80,000 in loans when I finished. So, I began to search for other schools with this degree for less.

Liberty University had the same degree for $27,000. It was a Christian School that I had considered attending for my Masters of Divinity. It turned out to be a better deal. If I added four more classes to my degree, I would be eligible in most states for a license to practice counseling. So, I said, "You know what God, I think this is where you're leading me." It's a Christian school which added the biblical worldview to our profession, which was a perfect match for me. The school was fully accredited, and the program was CACREP accredited and one of the top 4 online programs.

I started my master's in school counseling in January 2018. I remember him bragging about helping me make these decisions. I'm like, "Dude; you tried to talk me into going in the hole at NYU." But that's the kind of thing he would do: if something turned out great, he took the credit for it, and if it didn't, he would say I told them not to do that. He loved making those testimonies a part of his sermons.

This is why even though I was convicted about not going to church, I couldn't sit in the front row like everything was fine anymore. At that point, I had given up, and I was embarrassed that I had gotten so low that I didn't want to live anymore. I also know that I would go to church, and instead of getting anything, I was always pouring out. Even when I came in feeling low, I felt obligated to minister, lay hands, and pray for people. I couldn't help it. But, no more. I had nothing to give. Then he realized that our absence was causing attendance and finances to go down. Despite saying every week that he was sick as a dog, he found the strength to go because now our livelihood is being affected. He was extremely upset with me because I had been running everything for the past two years, and now he had to get up and do it himself. I realized that by doing everything for him, I was just enabling him. Now that I refused, he stepped up. It had been about a year that he wasn't showing up, but now he suddenly had some strength. Good for him.

The only problem is I don't know if that was good or bad. Now he was in the pulpit saying how sick he is all the time and that he has no support and nobody was helping. There was a time that I was home, and I got calls from some of the members saying that he told the congregation that he has spiders in his body and that is why he has Band-Aids on his head, and the world needs to know his story. He began to tell the people that he was the human Spider-Man and that no one believes him, but when he gets finished, the world would know that this is real. I didn't have any words for this. This is why I had no plans to return to the church. I'm not going to sit in the front and cosign this irrational behavior, nor am I going to try to explain to the congregation who have faith in him and God. If the people are smart enough to do their research, they will figure it out; but it won't be me that discourages them.

The day I knew that my husband was gone and probably not coming back was the day before Thanksgiving. He came home with all kinds of supplies from the drugstore, saying that the Holy Ghost showed him how to fix himself. The stool that we had sent to the doctors showed no parasites and no bugs in his body, so he figured the doctors did not know what they were talking about, and he dismissed them entirely. Therefore, he decided he was going to fix himself. I lived downstairs, so I didn't always see all of his concoctions and his experiments, but when you entered our master bedroom, it looked like a mad scientist/hoarder lived there.

So, on this particular day, I walked into the room, and there was a bit of a cloud in the air because he had been pouring powder used for lice on his genitals. He was mixing it with some creams and rubbing it over his testicles. He had all kinds of stuff in the bed with him, and he was lying down, rubbing it on himself, saying the Lord told him to do this, and it's working. He said the mothership was overtaking him in this area because I was supposed to cover that area, and I wasn't. The tears began to well up in my eyes. I said to him, "It's the day before Thanksgiving; what are you doing?" He said, "You just don't get it." When I saw him grab the Raid for spiders and spray it on his genitals, I was in total disbelief. I yelled, "What are you doing? That has got to be dangerous! That is a chemical!" I didn't know what it could do, but I knew it couldn't be right. He said, "Don't worry, it's coming out. This is about to be over." He always said that! He said that about the computers, then he said it about the worms.

Every week it was almost over, but it never ended. This had been going on for years now.

I cried and said, "I'm not going to do this with you. I am going to try and figure out what the children and I are going to do for Thanksgiving tomorrow." I had already decided we were not going to have a Thanksgiving at my house that year. It was too much stress for the family, and I couldn't host. My parents and family had already questioned why he never came downstairs for the past two years during holidays. For two years in a row, my mother came for an entire week and never saw him. Even though he was out preaching at the church some Sundays, the rest of the week, he was doing his experiments with his body, locked in the room. At this point, I started telling my family that he has a little anxiety and depression, and I'm just trying to see to it that he gets help and gets better. They had no idea the intensity of what I was going through, and I surely didn't tell them what I was battling and that I tried to commit suicide.

When I woke up that morning, I decided the kids, and I would go out to eat or find someone's house to visit. I went upstairs to check on him and see if he may have been well enough to join us. He started weeping, saying that his testicles were stuck to his legs and all burnt up. I looked at him and said, "Well, this is obvious if you were spraying yourself with Raid." The disgust with which he looked at me was piercing. He yelled at me for insinuating that he had done this to himself. He said that his testicles were burnt up because the spiders were defending themselves by shooting venom, which was burning his private areas. At that point, I was speechless. I offered to take him to the hospital, but he refused. I told him that I would bring him some food back, and the kids and I left.

At this point, I didn't think he was going to get better, so I started to look for positions as a teacher's assistant in the neighborhood. I found a school for the developmentally disabled one town over. The children at this school were mostly autistic, and I had worked with that population before. I went in for the interview, and because I had a bachelor's degree, I was top-tier as a teacher's assistant, making close to $16 hour and received a 3% raise a couple of months later. I hated leaving my children's school, but this was a full-time position with excellent medical and dental benefits. I felt good telling my husband that now he didn't have to pay $3000 in medical and dental insurance per month, but I could cover the whole family. I had to get my teachers assistant certification renewed. There was some goodness happening in my life, and I needed that. It had been so dark for so long, and I needed some light.

The job was not easy, but the students were rewarding. They were mute, violent at times, and I had to do takedowns. Sometimes they had accidents that had to be changed. It was okay because I was working towards something, and I had my own money. I was in school, so I knew this would only be temporary. The staff was mostly young students as DSP's, and at 40, this was taxing on my body.

Nonetheless, I was grateful to have a job. After toughing it out with the developmentally disabled, I had to come home to the mentally ill. I would come back looking forward to doing homework and taking care of my children, but would always walk into my husband's episodes.

One day I came home from work, and he had on a hazmat suit. I'm talking about suits similar to the one worn by agents in the movie E.T. with the glass front on the hood for quarantine. As I opened the door, he ran downstairs and said, "You gotta come see this!" He said there was stuff in the walls and ceilings, and he wanted me to see it. It was always dust or dark spots on the wall. He would always yell at me to look even when I was looking right where he was pointing. Then he said, "Look at me, look at how I'm sweating!" I reminded him that he had on a layer of clothing with a hazmat suit over it and that he should be sweating. He said he was sweating unusually and was frustrated that I "couldn't see." It was beyond arguing or rationalizing. I just said okay.

Then there were times he tried to convince me that we all had something in us.

One day he grabbed my 11-year-old son and pointed out a cut or scar he had on his arm and claimed that he was sick. He said, "But don't worry, I know how to get it out." I grabbed my son and said, "Don't you dare put your hands, concoctions, tools, or anything on my child. If he has anything, we will see a doctor." At that point, I didn't feel good about leaving the kids alone with him. He never paid them any mind, but I didn't want him to get any bright ideas while I was gone.

On top of everything else, I see that we are getting foreclosure notices as I'm checking the mail. He stopped opening the mail because he was consumed with getting the spiders out of his body. Seeing the foreclosure notice scared me because I didn't know what it meant. Will I come home and one day be locked out of our house? So, I started calling and researching what we could do. I started a process of modification. Now, I had to fight with him the year prior to get our taxes done to get my daughter and our second oldest into college. I had a fight again to get all the paperwork and all taxes done to modify the house. I learned a good lesson: not to let someone else control everything that concerns my life. I started keeping files and paperwork for myself. It took months to get paperwork that should have been in some sort of file or in a computer somewhere. It was like pulling teeth to get the bills paid around the house. Either way, I was getting it done the best I could.

It was rough, but I still managed to get all A's in school. I was working and taking care of the kids. The second eldest couldn't take all of the projects and yelling, and he decided to move down south with friends. I told him, no, but one day I came home, and he was packed to go. He said that his dad knew. I just let it go because if someone was able to get away from this madness, who am I to stop it? The handful of faithful friends continued to check in from afar because this situation was daunting and dark. I was glad to talk to sane people daily who made sure I remained balanced in the madness.

Frequently, when I would go out, he would question where I was. One day while I was out preaching, he called around and said, "Watch her because she will have you watching the kids and be out with a man." They had to tell him she's out preaching, and the saints are with her. Then he would yell at me, saying, "What are you going to do? Will you finish school, get yourself together, and leave me?" Well, at this point, I told him, "I want you to get yourself together. I have a mustard seed of faith that God is able. But not only have you been sick, but you have also been abusive, and no matter how much I try to help you, you've made me your enemy. I want to see you well, but if you don't get help eventually, I will get myself together and leave for my sanity. I shouldn't have to stay in this abusive relationship. I won't say what God can't do, but I just want you to get yourself together."

If I could be honest, there were times that he was so horrible that I ran off and slept in the park. I considered leaving him, but I had been a stay-at-home mom for ten years, I wasn't making enough money to go anywhere, and I didn't want to uproot my children from the way they were used to living, with nowhere to take them. For God's sake, we were Christians, and we were supposed to be able to work through anything! I didn't want to disappoint the church. Then I know he would tell people I left him sick, especially after he had been grooming everyone to believe I wasn't taken of him anyway. Plus, where would I go? I didn't want to live off of other people, so until I could support myself, I had to stay in this hell. This is what happens with some women who are being taken care of by an abusive man. Staying in an abusive situation is less scary than starting life over on our own. Oh, but how I would soon learn how staying longer than you should can be damaging or sometimes deadly!

Chapter 10
THE BEGINNING OF THE END

Now the abuse is so intense. There were times that I tried to speak up for myself just to regain my strength. But I knew when to speak up and argue and when to just back down. I kept trying to talk him into seeing a therapist, mainly at times when he would admit that something more than physical may be wrong with him. But, he could never fully admit it. I found different specialists that he could talk to in hopes that they would tell him what was going on. I researched hospitals, addiction recovery rehabs, bipolar, paranoid schizophrenia, and then narcissistic personality disorder (after one of our friends brought that to my attention).

At first, I adamantly denied the possibility of him being a narcissist (not fully knowing all of the traits) but, after learning them, I realized that even before the last four years of events, he had demonstrated signs of narcissistic personality disorder. When I brought any of this to his attention, it would just make him angry. It's crazy because, after that, he tried to tell me that I was the narcissist because I couldn't take his criticism of me or from anyone else. This is one of the first traits of being a narcissist: turning the story around and saying you are what they are clearly displaying. Then he tried to convince me that I was depressed because my single didn't do well, which was not true. After all, I was so proud of all I had done that year. He tried to make it seem like the single failed.

In his opinion, everyone was against him; the organization was against him. He hated me, and he would constantly say he gave me everything, and I gave him nothing. According to him, I was the worst wife in the world while he was the best husband that a girl could desire. Talking to friends, they helped me remember the truth: I was there, I was a rider, I built with him. I had to remind him of that every time he threw those darts because I refused to let those negative conversations sink to the point that I was depressed again. It was a battle, with depression trying to take over, but I had to keep pushing and fighting for my kids.

I kept asking God, "Why? God, why are you letting this happen like this? God, did I not pray and fast enough? God, what more could I have done?" And one day, God dropped the download. Your praying and your fasting are so that you can endure and learn how to gain strength through your trials. You can't make him do anything, even when you pray.

God let me know it was his pride that brought him this low and until he let down his pride and dealt with his issues he would remain. He had the "I" mentality, I did this, and I did that, everyone is against me because I.... He had forgotten who gave him the gifts and abilities.

That download changed the narrative for me. It was not my fault, and I wasn't responsible for changing him or fixing him. So, I'll keep my head up and keep pushing. I responded differently after this. So now it was, if I can, I will; if I can't, I won't. With this attitude, he said I was a cold narcissist. But, I had to survive. The truth is I should have walked away before I wanted to take my life, but as woman we are told to be loyal and faithful. In actuality, things had gone too far.

However, I didn't regret it. I knew I had done everything in my human ability as a wife to help him. I was done as a lover, but I was still a good human. Then we got the news that the Patriarch of the organization we were a part of had passed away. This was a man that he admired and looked up to. There was talk within the organization that it was more than a sickness that my husband was experiencing. People were saying that the Patriarch knew it, and told people to check in and see what was going on before my husband started telling people about the worms and spiders. He (the Patriarch) was sick and could not himself. Word got out that my husband was preaching about spiders in his body.

I knew that the news of this man's passing would affect him greatly. They were trying to gauge if he should speak at the funeral, and trying to assess if he would go off because at the last meeting he reportedly said some disturbing things. I told them it was their call. Well, they took a chance. And the whole time I was sick to my stomach; afraid of what he would say. It turns out I was right to be frightened. He said some things about the brothers being jealous of him, comparing himself as Joseph in the bible. He inferred that he was the beloved son with the coat of many colors and these men were the brothers that threw him in the pit. I was embarrassed, but I also knew it could have been worse. He truly believed that some of the other Bishops were jealous of him, but I started poking holes in those stories after a while. He had us warring with and against people for nothing. Don't get me wrong; it happens. I just don't know how much was real and how much was his delusion.

As the minister of music for the organization, I tried to get back in and become a part of the convocation, which was the next month. One of the days that I came home from convocation was the beginning of the end. I went to prayer day during convocation week. God knows I needed prayer. So, I hustled to get there (which was 1.5 hours away). I was so distracted trying to get there that I didn't realize I was low on gas and ran out and had to wait for AAA to bring me some. Now I was going to be late, but I didn't care. I just wanted to get to prayer. I had been in a struggle, and in twentysomething years of salvation, I wasn't going to church, which was not something I typically did. I arrived by the end of the service, and it was just what I needed, but then I couldn't get into the car and had to call AAA again for help to get into the locked vehicle.

The battery in the key had died. One of our members was so happy to see me, so she waited for all of this to take place. I had also promised to see one of our members who had been in the hospital for a week. This mother loved us so much, and I wanted to make sure I went to see her. I only stayed for a few minutes because her memory wasn't the greatest, but it was still good to see her. I had to find something white for the official day when I left her. I had no idea what I was getting ready to walk into when I got home. He started badgering me, asking where I had been and demanding that I give him my phone.

I didn't care and gave it to him. After asking questions about the locations of my phone pings, he started yelling. I believe this was because he didn't find what he was seeking. I told him to give me back my phone and grabbed it. At this moment, he reaches down, grabs my foot and lifted it, causing me to fall back; breaking the ottoman in our bedroom and landing on the back of my head. My daughter ran in, and he put on a gentle voice, saying, "Hey, mommy just fell." She said, "No, you just grabbed her leg and made her fall." I felt the back of my head to make sure it wasn't bleeding. I was in shock. He told my 6-year-old daughter to go back in the room while he took my phone and started smashing it with a hammer. At that point I left the room, grabbed some stuff, and decided to leave the house. I ran to the home of those who knew he was not well and they were very upset and disheartened, but not surprised. One of our male friends said, "Oh no, how bout I go there and have words with him?" This was the brother who had disappeared for some time. He was one that confronted my husband on things that he saw that was not right.

From that point on, my husband would plant seeds to us about his past, his character, and even to his own wife, which I could never understand, but I do now. This brother had already seen the narcissistic behaviors, he had seen the verbal abuse and had tried to warn his wife and those close to him, but my husband was so good with reminding you that he had been there for you and on your side that no one would dispute him when he spoke about others because he was the man of God and a powerful prophet.

So, this brother was ready to have words with him. We convinced him it was not necessary. It was a fight, but we succeeded. He told me that he could identify with where I was at this point. He also defamed this man's character to as many as he could. He knew what it felt like to be ostracized and manipulated by this man. It broke his heart to see me in the hospital knowing that the only way a person such as myself who always encouraged everyone else, and was so happy, fun, loving, and optimistic could get to the point where I didn't want to live was because of what my husband had done to me. And it was heartbreaking. He knew that it was time that everyone stopped tiptoeing around him because of his title and to deal with him as a man. But we all were still very sympathetic towards him, saying, "He is not mentally well," giving him a pass.

I stayed there overnight. I'm not sure if any of them spoke to him that evening, but the next day as they were on the phone with him, he was talking crazy, telling them where to find all of his essential paperwork and that he was going to burn the house down. He was speaking as if he was no longer going to be with us. This shook me because although I was sick of him and feeling so tired and hurt, I surely didn't want to see him kill himself. We all got in our cars from wherever we were and headed to him. One of the ladies got there before us, and also told his mother to get there because she could get there faster. As I am in route with one of the other sisters, we receive the call that I should not come. He was speaking so horribly of me and was accusing me of cheating. They didn't think it was safe for me to come. So, I stayed in a nearby store until the air was clear. It took so long; I decided to get back to my kids. He also had some very negative things to say about that brother, and it was decided that it was best that he not show up as well. Those ladies talked to him for hours, and it seemed like he was okay when they left. But the next day, he was at it again, and it seemed way more intense. Not knowing if we could get to him fast enough, they called the cops. I was notified and met them at the nearest Comprehensive Psychiatric Emergency Program (CPEP).

At the intake, they needed to speak to me to find out what was going on and for his medical history. It was a relief, but I was afraid. I wanted to tell them everything that was happening so that he could finally get the psychiatric help that he needed. I began to explain to them everything that occurred in the last four years, starting with the first panic attack in Virginia. I begged them not to tell him that I said this because he would be very angry with me. Next thing I know, there was a bed open at one of the psychiatric hospitals, and they sent him there. I cannot tell you the emotional roller coaster and battle that I endured that week. His mother was disgusted with me, saying it was my fault. He told them not to let me see him. I had been researching individual hospitals and was always trying to find him something peaceful on the water where he could recover. But this place wasn't one of those beautiful hospitals. I laid awake for those few nights, worried about his safety, if he was eating, and if he was okay. I even attempted to speak to the social worker who said she couldn't disclose anything to me because he would not allow it. But I just informed them that he came from a good home and was not just some guy off the street and asked her to please see to it that he's treated well. She couldn't disclose any information, but I could tell that she understood what was going on. He was so upset with me that I was unable to go to the hospital. I wasn't the one who called, but they had every right to take him to the hospital if he was expressing suicidal ideations.

Meanwhile, those that were close came around and said I should try to get the church back in place. They thought that this could all be a good thing because he may finally get the help that he needs. With the extended psychotic break, we thought the hospital might keep him for some time, especially since he was suicidal. So, I went to church. I didn't tell them anything, but I encouraged them to work with me to get the church back where it needed to be because it was dwindling. I was hoping to do that so that when he came home and was better, we could return to our lives before all of this.

I continued to call to get information, but they couldn't give me any. One day I called to see what was going on and was told that I might have to ask another family member about his discharge. He had only been hospitalized for seven days. I was back in my home, trying to get my children settled and get back to our lives. I remember being so scared. What did they mean? Was he coming home? Sure enough, the next thing I knew, he was pulling up to the house with his mother and his godmother. I went into my room and locked the door. I didn't even come out. I called the ladies that were with us through this ordeal to come over and help me to have this initial conversation with him. He was the worst. He was proud and arrogant. He said he was going to forgive us and that there was nothing wrong with him. He told us that the people at the hospital knew that he was sane and said to him that either your wife doesn't love you any more or is cheating on you. He told us the stories about his time there and how he was counseling all of the mentally ill patients there. He said they had become his friends. He then demanded that I quit my job and take care of him and the family like I was supposed to. The ladies and I interjected and reminded him that it was his attack on me and his suicidal ideations that led to his hospitalization.

I already knew that this was not going to be good. They left me here with him. All I remember is him telling me that I had to come to the bed because he was scared and had been through trauma at the psychiatric hospital. My sympathy led me to go up to the room, and I decided to sit up and sleep in the chair. He yelled at me, saying I was going to sleep in the bed. He even tried to force me to sleep with him. I told him, "First of all, it's been years since we slept together, and we would need a lot of counseling and help if that's even going to be the case." He yelled and screamed at me for the rest of the night. He accused me of sleeping with that brother and searched through my computers, my iCloud, etc. We always had each other's passwords. I watched him angrily, going through my things without care. He was getting so upset because he couldn't find anything, and he wanted me to confess. I told him I would not admit to what I did not do. He also said he was going to check my phone every day, and I told him that I refuse to live in prison. But there was no arguing with him. He would not let me sleep. I pleaded with him, reminding him that I had to go to work in the morning.

Every time I dozed off, he would start yelling louder. When the sun came up, I just got dressed and went to work.

When I got home from work, one of the ladies and his mother was in the garage; I guess working on another one of his projects. He was so enraged and was moving erratically like he always did. I remember saying I can't wait to go to bed. He gave me money and told me to get some ice and some food so that I could make dinner and feed the family. I didn't feel like arguing, so I went to the store for the food, came back and left it on the counter, and went to bed. I went into the room, and I plopped in that bed. I was exhausted. One of the ladies left to take his mother home, and when he came to my room and continued to accuse me of sleeping around. He started asking questions about the day we were all heading to help him. He was getting furious with my answers to his questions.

He jumped on top of me, and I started screaming, I looked over at the dumbbell that was next to me, and as I went to grab it, he grabbed it. I will never forget the rage on his face as he bashed it across my head. My head and face had a burning sensation. My son and my oldest daughter had run into the room, screaming. I jumped out of bed and ran downstairs. My children ran after me, and when they saw my face, they were screaming and yelling. My husband kept looking at me, saying, "What happened? What happened?" Then he grabbed a knife and said, "I'll just kill myself." My 10-year-old son had nightmares of his dad with a knife in his hand many times after that. I ran in the bathroom to call the pastor/lady/friend that took his mother home. When I looked in the mirror, the whole right side of my face was swollen. I asked her to come back, explaining that my husband had just hit me in the head with a dumbbell. I tried to take the kids and leave, but he would not let us go. At this point, it was really scary. He started getting upset about my older daughter standing at the bathroom door trying to protect me. He said, "I know that's your mom, but I have taking care of you more than your mom and dad for most of your life."

That lady returned quickly and was shocked at the condition of my face. I told her I wasn't answering the questions that he was asking the way he wanted. I asked her to explain the situation to my husband because she was there. He then proceeded to tell her that I had an emotional relationship with the brother in question. He had been encouraging me, calling me like everyone else this entire year, making sure that I was okay. And he took those encouraging messages and told her that I was having an emotional affair with him. He started screaming, yelling, and pacing back and forth in the house. He didn't want us to leave, and he seemed unstable.

We sent the kids to the basement so that they didn't have to witness or hear this traumatic behavior. After about 6 hours of trying to calm him down, he attempted to take pills and lay in his bishops' regalia and die. He ranted about me being a bad wife, him being a wonderful husband, and all of the sickness that he had to endure. He was crying, but then he would yell and become raging which was scary. I told this sister, "Why don't we just grab the kids and try to get out of here?" He then commenced to saying that he was going to kill me, that brother, the kids, and then himself. This was super scary. It was the most traumatic experience I ever witnessed. That sister had to go to therapy after this experience, and so did me and my children.

He started praying and crying, and around 2 am, he looked at me with this weird facial expression like he had just gotten a download from the Holy Ghost. Then he said, "The Holy Ghost just showed me it's not just emotional; you are having a full out affair with that brother."

He jumped up, ripped my wedding rings off my fingers, and told me I had five minutes to get out of his house. I tried to grab my pocketbook and the children, and he ripped my pocketbook off of my back. He told me that I was leaving with nothing; that he had given me all of this and I could take nothing with me. We grabbed those kids and ran out so fast. We started driving and we didn't stop until I was at my mother's house in Brooklyn. When my mother saw my face, she was in disbelief and she called my father right away. When my father got to the house and saw my face, he started crying. He said, "You are my only child. If something was to happen to you, I'd have no one."

My mother told me to go back to my home and called the police. My dad said, "If you do not call the police, then I'm going to have to take matters into my own hands. It doesn't matter if he is a bishop, he should not have put his hands on you. And he needs hand put on him."

From the time I left the house, my husband was sending me text messages in a group text with that young lady. They were disgusting. He said if I told anyone that he had hit me, he was going to lie and say that it was my boyfriend that hit me. He told me in those text messages to not even try to get child support for the kids because he didn't want anything to do with them or me. He said if I told people that he hit me and if I tried to come after him, when he gets finished tarnishing my name and telling the world what a horrible person I am, I'll never be able to show my face anywhere. He said that the next time when I tried to commit suicide, after he gets finished destroying and defaming my name, I would make sure that it was complete. He literally stayed up all night sending me over 40 pages of text messages. The messages didn't stop coming until we pulled up to the house with the cops at 2pm. That young lady told me to stop reading the messages, and for the first time she recognized and admitted that I was in an abusive relationship and it had to stop today. We had to go back to the house with the police, and they took him and arrested him. He tried to play as if he didn't know what had happened. He said I'm an Archbishop, and my dad said, "And an archbishop shouldn't hit his wife."

I will probably never forget this event in my life because he was arrested the day before his birthday. I remember sending him a message the next morning on his birthday. One of the counselors at the police station told me to make sure that I was at the courthouse to get a restraining order, or else he could come back home and kill me. So, I went there and met with the counselor, and she went into the court asking for a restraining order. I was so relieved because I didn't know what he would do once he came home. The people at the church called me to tell me that he called in and asked to be put on the speaker and said to them that the devil was after him, but he's going to be vindicated. I don't know why he brought the church into this because I wasn't planning on telling them. I still didn't want to tarnish his name because I thought maybe if he ever got better, he would be able to stand up and continue to fulfill his purpose. But that was me continuing to cover him when he could care less about me.

As soon as he got home, he texted the crew and started talking about me and this brother like a dog. He told everyone that he hired a private investigator and had all this evidence against us, which was untrue. He was now not only paranoid and out of his mind, but was making up stuff as he went. I think the court ordered him to see a counselor. One day he called me and said, "Listen, let me come back home. I saw a therapist, and it wasn't you. My mom was an alcoholic, and the traumatic events happening to me growing up...my grandmother always telling me to be a good boy because she didn't have to take me in messed me up. So, I always tried to be good to everyone. Please let me come back home, and we can work this out." I was happy to hear that he was getting counseling. And I do believe that his traumatic childhood may have been the root of this mental breakdown along with other factors such as genetics and addiction issues in his lineage.

However, I did not want to lose the peace that I was getting with that man not being in the house. There was no way I was letting him back in the house and especially not after one or two counseling sessions. Considering the last four years of insanity that my children and I had to suffer through, we needed more than a couple weeks. He should have been forced to get help a long time ago. And when I told him he could not come home, he became furious and started yelling at me angrily again. So, I hung up the phone and blocked him. Then his mother called me and said she needed to come and get his medicine because he is very sick. Now, after she was mean and mad at me, knowing that he was mentally ill, I allowed her to come and get his medicine. She then called me again a week later and asked that she go and get some more of his stuff. Keep in mind that he was supposed to come one time with the police to grab some of his belongings. But he didn't want to do that. So, I let her come in, and from what I saw, all she left with was some of his computers and his Range Rover. Despite it all, I was still nice.

Now he is telling people that I lied and said he hit me, called me all kinds of whores to people and telling them whatever he could think up. So, when his mom called me again to get more of his things, I said, "No, tell him to come with the cops and get what he can get and then leave me alone." He wanted me to leave with nothing, he wanted me to have nothing, and he wanted me to have no one. The trap that he set for me has come upon him. His plot and plan didn't work.

When that brother found out what had happened to me and the things that my husband was saying, he wanted to get at him. He called him and told him if a real man had a problem, he would step to a real man and not hide behind text messages. He lit into him a few times. He saw a lot of stuff but never said anything except to those close to him, and he tried to respect God in this man and his title. But at this point, he had had it. He was no longer acting like a man of God and did not deserve to be treated as such. See what we all came to realize, even with the mental illness, that there is still a smart, calculated and manipulative man working through it. This brother was the first of us, even before the breakdown, to call him out. This is the reason my husband already hated this man so much. So, this was a perfect plot to take two people that he hated down at once.

This brother had never spoken negatively about my husband to me. He knew I was loyal. But after this situation, the things that he began to share with me that my husband had planted seeds even in his marriage, something that he would say about him to his wife, I couldn't believe. But then again, I watched how he had done it with others, so it all makes sense. The same way he did it with the workers at the church, the same way he did it to me, he did the same thing with couples. I have many that can attest to that today. Many didn't realize while it was going on, but when they look back the way he used to play people against each other, they now can see. The thing about this brother was that he was the one person who no longer cared about the title and spoke up. It was really good to have a conversation with someone who understood the calculation, and the very intricacies of his narcissistic ways. If you don't know anything about narcissists again they work intricately, in very subtle ways. You don't know you're being abused, and you don't realize how much damage is done to you mentally until you begin the process of healing. You don't realize how much they have infiltrated your mind and made you believe terrible things about yourself. There is PTSD involved because you are traumatized, afraid to make decisions, and unsure of yourself because of all of the negative seeds planted by them. They also make people around them believe in them and love them so that they will trust and believe what they say about others.

This brother began to share some of those feelings he had when working with him years back. He said that's why he had to get away from it all. I had no idea that's why he stopped coming around. I always wondered. He began to share with me that me being down-to-earth and cool and always so compassionate with people, helped balance out our ministry. He said he hated bullies because he was bullied as a child, and if I didn't have anybody else to stand up, he had my back. Honestly, I began to feel safe, but more importantly, like I wasn't crazy for what I knew had taken place. Even with all that had transpired, everyone was still tiptoeing around him and not outright telling him about himself. Don't get me wrong; there was no getting through to him. Conversations with him left you with a headache, but I believe people were still trying to respect the title when he had already disrespected it himself.

We allowed this renegade behavior and created a monster for covering and not speaking against wrong. Sadly, when it's so calculated and subtle, some stuff went unnoticed. We all also had a respect for God and his leadership. However, when a man is abusive, disrespectful, and arrogant, we no longer should have to respect the disrespectful. Nor do we have to agree with something if it's wrong. I pride myself in getting to know people for myself and not what people said. This is why he said I was siding with his enemies. Husband, Bishop, and all, if he said something that didn't sit right with me (not that I always caught it), I questioned it. Maybe I questioned it privately, but I still questioned it.

Now that he was gone, it made me look at the entire course of our marriage and question everything. Was this real? Was this manipulation? Was that even genuine? Did you do anything from your heart? Although it was a shaky start, I locked into forever with this man. I was afraid to, but I did. Ministry and marriage were the end game, and I was in for the long haul. I felt like I should have remained guarded to save myself from this pain, but here begins the healing process, which starts with cleaning up the rubbish from the disaster, working through my choices, and what occurred.

Chapter 11

REBUILDING: THE HEALING PROCESS BEGINS

While the healing process was beginning, I had no other choice but also to begin the process of rebuilding. I was rebuilding after I tried to commit suicide but was in limbo about my marriage. Now I must rebuild without a husband and a church. I was trying to get used to this new peace that I had. I didn't have to walk in on him, cutting his body open; I didn't have to come home to all the yelling and negativity. With him, I never knew what I was going to go home and see or experience. Now it was just me and my two babies-- all love. Those who he had been talking to had already seen the mental breakdown, so I didn't care how much he lied to them about me. At this point, everything he was saying was a lie. I don't know what he was putting his poor mother through over there, but I was glad it was her and not me. Now, after she has accused me of neglecting him, she would see what it is like to live with him every day.

The Day I Committed Suicide

Well, the little bit of peace that I thought I was engulfing upon, yet again, was coming to an end. After multiple calls and conversations, he decided that because he was not getting what he wanted, he was going to torment me further. He still wanted to come home, but that was not safe for the children and me, and with witnesses, on the phone, he was still angry and mentally unstable. He tried to talk about a plan to take care of the kids, but every conversation ended with him yelling and degrading me. So, there was no chance of negotiations. I would no longer let him disturb my peace.

One day he decided to go on Facebook all day long. He was posting silly jokes. This continued for about 24 hours. Everyone was laughing at first, but then someone asked him, "What are you doing, Bishop? Are you crazy?" After a while the jokes weren't making much sense. Of course, he got upset up with that question and wrote, "If you think I'm joking, if you think I'm crazy if you think something is wrong with me, meet me at prayer on Wednesday night at the church."

Now he has an audience because people realize something is wrong. He's continuing to rant and rave, and people are trying to find out what's happening. I ignored phone calls and what everyone was telling me. On Wednesday night, in October 2018, I start getting calls that he was losing it at the church. He told everyone that I was a terrible wife and that I was cheating with a couple of people, and even began to talk about my private parts to the people that came to the church. Now Wednesday night services usually had low attendance, but because of his Facebook rantings, people came out of the woodwork. His best friend (my big sis) had been hurt by him but was still worried about him and decided to go so she could pray with him. But he was saying such derogatory things that the pastors, this sister, and some other ministers and friends that came by to pray tried to get him to stop. He refused and he asked some of the security and ushers to physically remove the people who were trying to get him to be quiet, including his best friend. To this day she expresses how that experience scarred and hurt her. He continued from the pulpit, telling and exposing people's business. And he realized that some of the people were trying to put others out of the church just to cover him so that he would not be seen like this.

From what I heard, it was a horrific scene. He got so upset that he left the building, got in his car, and went live on Facebook. And he began to repeat the things that he was saying in the church. He then started talking about the organization, telling their business. People were afraid because he was going LIVE on social media and out driving on the road. He seemed unstable as if he was getting ready to go and do something stupid. People were afraid because of the way he was talking about me, hoping that he wasn't heading to do something to me. As he called out names, anytime people tried to call him to ask where he was and what he was doing, he commenced to telling their personal business, so now no one wanted to stop him. My phone was going off; my inbox was pinging all night. I told them that I didn't know where he was going or what he was doing.

Now I am terrorized and traumatized, not knowing what's going to happen next or what lies he's going to tell people. New lies were coming up, but with some of the things he was saying, I thank God some people could witness that he was lying. However, the church still didn't know the whole story, the church world that followed us via social media had no idea that this man had lost his mind for the last three years because I covered it so wonderfully.

People are trying to figure out if he's out of his mind or if this a breakdown because his wife betrayed him. I had bishops calling me asking how to find him. It didn't look like it was going to end well. For the next 24 hours, everyone had logged in to see my husband having a nervous breakdown on Facebook live. He also went live to show them how he had spiders coming out of his face, which of course, exposed his mental illness to those that were up in the wee hours in the morning.

He also accused me of sleeping with the person who helped me produce my music single. I was very good friends with him and his wife, and they are a very prominent couple in our community. So not only is he destroying his life, he's trying to destroy the lives of other families. He hated me making music, so he accused me of sleeping with my music producers. I had to call them and their family members to apologize and let them know he was not well. I wondered if there was something more that I could have done more to make him get help, especially since others outside of my circle are now being hurt. But I don't know what else I could've done.

Everyone kept telling me, don't say anything; don't lash out. A couple of the bishops and pastors went to search for him. I decided to make a statement on my page. I stated; this is not a show or a game, but what I had been suffering through for the past four years, and I asked them to pray for my family.

Some of our people were trying to figure out how to shut his page down because he was just exposing any and everybody that he could, saying whatever he wanted to about them. It was so upsetting, and this is what I had been trying to protect them from all these years by not saying anything. It was hurtful and embarrassing to me, but he also was making himself and our church look bad. Our church was shocked and broken-hearted. This was too much to bear, and no one could stop him.

He even talked about my mom and my dad on Facebook, saying that I said terrible things about them. He told everyone that he was staying with his mother, and while he was sleeping in the bed with his mom, he turned around and looked at her and tried to choke her because he thought she was me. That just let me know that I could never be in the same space with him again.

Not only was he going live, but YouTube bloggers were also taking clips of his lives and making news stories out of it. And of course, they take whatever he's doing and put their spin on it. I contacted one of the bloggers and asked him to please take it down because these are real human lives that they are making fun of and adding their spins to his wild stories. He didn't take it down, but he tried to humanize the situation and asked people to pray for our family. Another YouTube blogger asked me to come on his show and do an interview, but I had never been through anything like this, and I surely did not want to continue to publicize one of the biggest embarrassments of my life. The truth was, the bloggers only confirmed that he was not mentally well. Meanwhile, I was still trying to protect his image by not saying anything.

Why did I always want to protect him when it seemed that he could care less about protecting me?

People kept asking if I was okay because they were afraid for my life. Others felt that if even I did do all of the things he was saying, he did not have to air it out on social media. Either way, I just hated that we were the talk around our community. With both of us having 5000 followers on Facebook, many people knew us in the New York area, and we were the gossip of the city right now. I hated it. I don't think people understand the trauma of your business being spread all over social media. When you have a whole community in your personal space as I did, it was traumatizing.

At this point, anxiety and PTSD were imminent for me and everyone whose name was involved. Every time somebody called me to tell me that he posted something, I got headaches, and my stomach would be sick. He could make up any story and post it, and there was nothing I could do about it. I even went to the police to see if there's something they could do, and they told me just to turn off my social media. It's not that simple when you are a public figure in your community, though.

I never went LIVE, I never clapped back, and I didn't take interviews. One or two bishops called me when he first lost it on Facebook. I told them that if they believed they could talk him into getting help, they should. Another told me I should get the board to vote for him to be sat down until he gets help and we hold the church down. I was like, "Nope; I'm traumatized and hurt; therefore, I can't run the church again. Also, he is insane and abusive, sitting him down will not restrain him which means I could possibly have to deal with him coming to the church to fight me or kill me. No, thank you." Our trustees and board were the crew, and they had left as I'm sure they didn't want to deal with any more trauma.

I was in a twilight zone. I had been through a lot. I was going to take a break from classes because I would have anxiety just going to my computer and when I finally had the strength to get to the work, I would sit there, unable to organize my thoughts or keep them together. I spoke to that brother, who I now consider to be one of my closest friends, and he encouraged me to continue and finish strong. He said, "You can't let him win nor let this situation get the best of you. Be the strong, resilient first we know you to be". I spoke to my professors and told them what I had been enduring and what happened just before the semester started (the attack). They gave me 4 more weeks to complete my work, and I made it through the semester. What I thought I could not do, was done. That is when I understood how who is in your life at certain seasons is essential. Had I taken a semester off; honestly, I probably would not have gone back. I felt at this point if I could make it through the semester with the trauma that I had just endured, I can make it through any semester after that. It wasn't the A's that I was getting when I started; however, the B's didn't look that bad on my transcript either.

For Thanksgiving, I decided just to go and spend it with the kids' godparents to get away from everything. Even living all the way down South, this couple checked in and made sure the kids were okay. They sent school supplies and so much more. God was so gracious to keep those who I needed in my corner, who knew even without me asking when to call, and when I was in need. I saw my uncle while I was there, and they told me to move down there where I could give my kids the same quality of life they had in NY at literally half the price. For a single mother doing everything alone, that was enticing. But I had unfinished business in NY. After a wonderful time, it was back to real life.

Now I had been driving the Escalade the entire marriage because I was the one that did all the shopping and drove the five children around. Every couple of years, we would upgrade. It was the only car that could fit all of the kids. It was known that was my car, especially since the first Escalade was bought by trading in a vehicle that was in my name that I had paid off. At this point, registration was expired on the Escalade, and the insurance had lapsed. So, I called the insurance company and purchased insurance, which was easy because I had already been on the policy. I found the title for the Escalade and went to reregister the car. I was told that I could not register because the insurance had lapsed four times in a row. I thought, "Oh God, not another thing." I could not register the car for 45 days, but I had to turn in the plates while I waited.

So, I did. He had already taken the Range Rover, so I had to drive the two-door car, squeezing my children in there to get around. The only problem was that the registration on that car had expired also. I did not have insurance on that car and could not afford it because I already paid for the insurance on the Escalade. Although this was not okay, it was the only thing I could do to get to work and get my children to school. And I thought to myself, "Well, it's only 45 days."

While I was waiting, he decided to finally use his one time to come with the cops to get his things. There was a U-Haul and some of the brothers from our church knocking on my door with police. That man came into the house, and I could see that look in his eyes. He was still not well and moving and talking fast like a person who was high. He had been trying to ask me for our Escalade. And I had said no because that car was me and the kids' car. I also found out he owed $7,000 on the Range Rover and they repossessed it. He wasn't slick. He wanted the Escalade because it was the only car that we had that didn't have any more payments.

They wouldn't let him take the Escalade because it had no plates on it, and the registration was due. Either way, that was the only thing he came for because he wasn't taking anything else but a TV, a desk, and a few other things. He was yelling, "Where's my bishops' jewelry? See, I told y'all they are stealing from me!" His guys then found what he said was stolen. He kept trying to pull the officers aside to get them to let him take the car; I heard one of the officers say, "I see how you are bossing and pushing all these other guys around; telling them what to do and where to go, but that's not going to work on us. That car cannot leave this property without plates and registration. Y'all work that out in court."

After a while, the police were getting fed up with him and his behavior, especially after he started cursing me out and calling me a whore in front of my children. After cursing me out, they made him leave, while the brothers asked if they could stay and collect the rest of his things. I very nicely told them that it was not okay, and that I had been through enough torment and embarrassment, and the longer they stayed in my house, the longer the torment continued. They graciously began to leave.

Unbeknownst to me, my confidantes and closest friends were having a conversation about getting out here so that I can have someone with me while I was here feeling overpowered and bullied. That brother was the first to roll up on the scene prepared to stand with me. Thank God it was shortly after my husband was escorted out. God knows that would have been a scene. I'm not sure what he said to the brothers that were there, but he had worked with them previously, so it seemed like a cordial conversation, and everybody drove off peacefully. Shortly after, my big sis showed up with her husband. While we sat and talked about the manipulation and the pain he caused every last one of us over the years, it made me very sad. Periodically people would talk to me about things that he did to put people against each other. Even her husband who was not a part of the church began to share with me things I had no idea about. Why would he turn husbands against wives and wives against husbands? I'll never understand this.

This is not to expose him, but to expose this behavior. We were all street and book smart. We all had intuition or what the church describes as the Holy Ghost. It didn't matter, as we were still victims of this manipulation and emotional abuse. Some things were noticed, but somethings passed because we respected God and the God we thought was in him. He was able to take our flaws and faults to make people fight amongst each other and to trust and have more faith in him then their faith and trust in their spouses.

I got a call that he was going live on Facebook again, telling people that he came to the house, that we were stealing his stuff, that we had been hacking him for four years, and that my boyfriend came to protect me. I was so embarrassed by his lies and deceit. I had so much anxiety. I thought that since he was out of the house, I would be free from the torment, but he used social media to torment me every chance he got. I was so fed up with his behavior that I snapped. I searched my phone and found the pictures of my face from when he hit me with the dumbbell and posted them on Facebook. I explained in my post that I had been going through torment and abuse for many years, but I covered him while also trying to get him help. I said that he was not mentally well, but he is still calculated in what he was doing; that I had had enough and that after this, I would say no more.

When I put those pictures up, the response was enormous. Not only were people sending encouraging messages and praying for me, but some women began to confess that they were in abusive relationships, and others began to testify about how they got out. Other women were applauding me for speaking up because most women wouldn't because of his status. The disheartening part was that women were inboxing me who were married to pastors and ministers and were presently in abusive relationships and didn't know how to get out, but felt encouraged by me standing up. I didn't know what I was doing by putting up those pictures. Still, the overwhelming encouragement that other women were getting made me realize that I was in another situation that wasn't just for me but will eventually be a blessing for somebody else.

Having been raised by my mom and grandmother to be a strong, powerful woman, I was humiliated to have been attacked. After I put the pictures up, I had second thoughts. It's embarrassing that I let a man beat me. Although I wasn't being beaten every day, I was emotionally abused for years. When those women started to reach out to me, that is when I knew that I had to tell my story to help other women. There are many women in influential marriages, that are being abused, feeling less than, and don't know how to get out. As a counselor and a survivor, I knew it was my duty to lean in and figure out how to help others through my testimony. But not right now because I had so much on my plate, so much to get through, and so much to evaluate, heal, and come through—such as; he's still preaching, and every sermon is about this slew of enemies that he has, with me at the top of the list. He's there some Sundays and other Sundays he's suffering from "Lyme Disease." Oh yeah, this is the new disease he allegedly has.

Nonetheless, when he was there, I was the topic of the day. Therefore, the bullying, torment, and lies continued. No matter how much I have blocked him and his pages, people still tell me about it or inbox me about it. Everyone that was his friend, he disposed of. His theory is that the world was against him and the obsession with that is another clear symptom of paranoid schizophrenia. It was another way to gain sympathy and to take people's eyes off of his wicked ways.

The problem was he's still convincing a few people that he was legit, or they just felt sorry for him. But to post these Facebook live videos only further embarrassed him and my family. I don't think people realized how my five kids and I were tormented and embarrassed by this situation, and every time someone went live on Facebook with him preaching about us, they were a conduit to this continued pain for the kids and me. My kids' friends and family were following us as well, and they had to try to explain this catastrophe.

When I put my pictures up and began to explain what I had been going through with him, one of his sisters called me and sympathized, saying, "Why didn't you call us and tell us that you were going through this?" She told me, "You shouldn't have had to go through this by yourself. We have two uncles who have paranoid schizophrenia." I didn't know how to receive this information. I knew before the Adderall; he had symptoms of depression and anxiety. His mom also would have lots of stomach aches and irritability, which I believed were signs of anxiety. This would also explain her struggle with alcoholism (studies show mental health issues often lead to drug and alcohol abuse to ease those symptoms). So, I believed he inherited that. However, studies show that the long-term use of high doses of Adderall can cause delusions, hallucinations, and paranoia. The question was if this came from the overuse of this drug, or was this prone to happen due to genetics.

When I tried to call a lawyer to sue our family doctor for giving him all of these mixtures of high doses of psychotropic drugs, they all told me that it takes too much money to prove that a drug caused mental illness. Most times, there is a mental illness present, and the drugs only advance it. I'm assuming that is the case here. It could be drugs, or it could be genetics. At this point, I was done trying to figure out what was wrong with him. It was time to begin taking care of my children and the healing process for us.

I was receiving the letters about the house being in foreclosure. I had no idea what that meant because although I had maintained apartments on my own before, I never had to maintain a house on my own. I continued to make calls and do my research. He had the lights turned off on me, but I was able to put them in my name and pay that bill on my own. I had trouble with the gas bill, and after calling five times, I was able to get that bill in my name and start paying that from scratch. For a few days, the gas was off, and my children and I had to bathe using water that we heated in the microwave. I couldn't use my washing machine or my stove. You don't realize how much you need these utilities until they are gone. This is the stuff that I could have been going live about on Facebook while he continued to claim to be an innocent victim.

I continued to drive a car with no insurance and no registration until the 45 days were up. I went to register the vehicle and was told that there was a new title ordered, and it went to the address of the owner. What a bastard he was. He knew that the children and I needed a car, but ordered a new title, knowing it would go to his new address, so that I couldn't register our vehicle.

Money was so tight, so it was time to do what's best for the kids and me without worrying about his feelings. I decided to file for child support because why should I have to take care of the children by myself and struggle.

He was shocked because I had the kids' godfather with me. He showed up to court that day but couldn't stay calm for long. He yelled that I opened eight phones in his name, which is another insane claim. He became irate until the police on duty had to make him leave my presence. He never showed up to the next few court dates, so it went into judgement; in which support was due weekly. He paid a total of 4 or 5 payments, owing over $17,000 in child support at this point and still going. So even when you try to fight in court for this, it doesn't matter if a person chooses not to pay. It makes it even worse when they're a pastor who can hide all of the money they have coming in, no longer writing his own checks; therefore the city cannot garnish his wages. He also would not file taxes. Again, this was just more deception and manipulation. And he had the nerve to tell people that he was paying child support.

The struggle was getting real, so I started to apply within my company for managerial positions. They had great benefits that I did not want to lose. A couple of them never really came through, and that was discouraging also. But finally, a counseling position came through, working at the Office of Mental Health portion of our company, doing counseling, preparing treatment plans, and working to integrate the mentally ill back into the community. I enjoyed this position immediately. One, because this was my educational background, and also what I was presently in school for, and these were patients that knew they had an illness; however, they complied with their medications, and their treatment plans to maintain and to be better. This boosted my faith because, within a year, it was a promotion and a substantial raise. Not bad for a woman who was a stay-at-home mom for ten years. My bosses said that it was not just my experience, but it was my nice demeanor and understanding of working with the mentally ill.

Now I'm driving back and forth to this job where I have some of the best and the nicest staff. Two women begin to tell me their testimonies of going through foreclosure, and one had to deal with a narcissist who made her life a living hell. But what they said to me that it takes a few years before, you will have to leave your home and to keep checking in on the status of my house. That was a relief because all I needed was time to rebuild so I can stand on my own two feet. I was not ready to pull them out of school, from the environment of having their rooms and space in this gated community, which was safe for someone like me who's a single mom. My neighbors were so gracious to get my children to school in the morning because I had to leave for work before they had to get to their bus stops. At this point, I would have to move out of state to give them this type of life as a single parent. New York is tough for single moms or dads.

I had been driving the car for six months with no registration, no insurance, and it could be repossessed at any moment. It was so risky, but I didn't know what else to do because I needed to work so that my kids and I could live. My friends worried about me being on the road like that. After a while, one of my friends who buys and sells cars at auctions told me that I could get a decent car for cheap and fix it up so that I could still have something to go back and forth to work. I still had to come up with a lump sum for that car, so I had to let down my pride and ask for help. I was living from paycheck to paycheck, but I knew I needed to do something when I was almost hit head-on by a car. I couldn't continue to drive without insurance. My kid's godfather and that brother, helped me to get money for a used car and to get it fixed to be on the road.

I decided that I shouldn't have to beg and borrow for money when these children have a father who is living somewhere responsibility free. He still had the church, and that church is no longer paying the housing allowance; therefore, he controls all of the finances, keeping them to himself. Whether he's collecting a salary or not, he is not thinking about taking care of his children or the responsibilities he left behind. Although he seemed out of his mind with the talk about spiders and enemies all the time, he was still bright and smart enough to know how to play the court system, to know how to have people thinking that he just wants to come and get the Escalade, to move around from place to place and change addresses not to be served in court. Just because they are mentally ill doesn't mean they're not still smart. I would chalk everything up to his mental illness, but most times, he knew exactly what he was doing.

Meanwhile, my faith is reeling, the hustle was real, and trying to maintain my mental health was work. Remember, I no longer had a church home now, and the awkwardness of trying to walk into places where people knew me and even places where no one knew me was always a struggle. I started to watch TD Jakes every Sunday, and my God, it was better than going into some of these Sunday morning services. I was now strengthened to carry on for the week. I was still asking God why it had to go this way, and he kept telling me because of the plan and purpose of my life. He continued to let me know he could trust me with this plan, and with this purpose. I just remember crying out of 2018 into 2019 on New Year's Eve.

I cried so hard; it was like a purge. I was beginning the process of letting it go. When I walked in the door on New Year's Eve, my oldest daughter was home, and so were my two little ones. I told them I loved them and couldn't stop crying from the car until I saw them. And they hugged me and started crying with me. It was like they knew why I was crying and/or they were purging with me. We had been through so much. Although I sheltered them from 2014 to 2017, they saw and experienced way too much in 2018. However, this healing would be ongoing. As for my children, I continued to do mental health checks and talk to them about our experience in a healthy and age-appropriate manner. Most times we mess up by telling kids hush or sweeping things under the rug like nothing ever happened. I refused to continue this cycle in our culture with my children.

Chapter 12

FREEDOM/THE HEALING PROCESS CONTINUES

As I began a new journey of consecration and prayer, I wrote a song called "I Am Enough," which was birthed from a headliner about a well-known music artist who had been abusing young women. I wondered, "Why did these women feel they had to walk into situations for fame and fortune? Why did they allow this man (because they were not kidnapped), to treat them in this way?" This man was also someone who wined and dined them and initially treated them well; promising them fame. He then began to mentally break them down and abuse them, and they didn't even want to leave the abusive situation. I could have been one of those girls. When I was 17 or 18, I loved this artist so much that I cried at his concert. I was a young singer and could have easily fallen into this same trap. However, I did fall into an abusive relationship. It may not have been as severe, but it was the same narrative. Then I said, "if we knew who we were if we knew how special we were, if we knew our value, beyond who we were in a relationship with, we would not allow people to treat us a certain way. If we knew that we were great with or without a man, we would not allow them to treat us like trash." Hence came my song.

While in transition, I touched base with a young branding consultant who was boosting his business. He connected with me via social media, asking if I had any advertisement needs. At the time, the handful of people were reminding me of the ministry on my life and how I had to get back to it. In my refusal, I decided I wanted to get back to just making my music. I knew I had to get busy to not fall back into depression, and I knew I

had to do what God called me to do, so I decided to start with music. I expressed to this young man my desire to pursue music again. I shared my experiences with mental health issues in my personal life and with my family, saying how much I would love to bring awareness to not only the church but the African American community. I told him that I might need his assistance for a book cover because I was challenging myself to tell my story.

I may not have clapped back on social media; I may not have made it my business to go around and defend myself against all the harmful lies that my husband was spreading about me, but this thing plagued my mind and my heart daily. It bothered me. I knew that there were plenty of people in our lives, and outside of my story that had been through a similar experience. As I began the process of healing, I realized I was not a horrible person. Talking to friends and family members who never wanted to speak up on what they had seen me going through before the mental illness also freed me.

I had family members who said, "I never liked his chauvinistic ways and how he used to talk to you." I had congregants that began to speak up and tell me some of the things that were done to them and how they noticed the way that he treated me as well and didn't like it. I began to think about the musicians and others who left the church and were hurt, maybe even feeling like they were not enough because of all of the damaging things he had said to them from the pulpit and in meetings. I called the musicians after everything happened to tell them they were excellent, and let them know that I thought we were such a great team and no matter how much he said that they weren't good enough, they were great. There were plenty of people that told me that we had one of the baddest bands in the city. Not only did I want to heal, but I wanted to see that others who endured this abuse knew that they were loved, and enough.

At this point, I decided to work on some old music that I had and figured that maybe I could do an EP with the new song as well. I wanted to write a book. I had always wanted to write the story of my life, but I had no idea the chapters would end this way. It didn't hurt to research to find out what it would take to begin writing my book. I decided just to start writing. People were telling me to write a book, leaving prophecies in my inbox without me ever making the announcement that I was writing, which was the confirmation that it was the plan. It encouraged me to keep going even when there were times that I wanted to stop.

Another monumental road to freedom was cleaning out my master bedroom and bathroom. That room had three or four tool chests that belonged in the garage. There were boxes and boxes of gadgets everywhere. Another sign that my husband also had OCD was that he had at least 20 of everything, no exaggeration. Twenty cameras that he put all around the house. Thousands of pens. So many cords for so many different gadgets inboxes. In my closet and bathroom, you couldn't see the counters or shelves. I had a friend come over who was a mental health professional and agreed that this was definitely the scene of someone who wasn't well. I started putting my clothes back in my walk-in closet, and I was able to see my bedroom as a bedroom again, and I cried. This room was traumatic for me, but if I was going to live here for a little while longer, I should have a place of peace to walk into each day and night. I prayed and consecrated in my room and asked God to help cleanse and clear all of the trauma that occurred in that space. The truth was that staying here was okay temporarily, but while I am here, I will be cleaning up my credit so that I can purchase my place of peace. That house was too big, and there was still too much trauma here. Plus, it was in foreclosure.

After some time, I decided to reach out to this young branding consultant about my book and my music. He reminded me that my husband and I both preached at his family's church. He said he admired us from afar. He reminded me that in spite of what I had been through, the ministry on my life wasn't over and was stronger now. He told me that looking from the outside; there were people out there who still loved me and were waiting for me to fulfill my purpose.

They needed my testimony and what God placed in me. It was one thing to hear it from people I called my confidantes and friends, but now to hear from those who watched from afar was even more affirming. He was one of many who confirmed this.

He asked what happened with the woman at the well. I began to express the message I had been preaching for years: there was a woman who was a low-class citizen, who had been married five times, and the man that she was living with was not her husband. In that context, women were already low-class citizens, and if they were not married, they had no voice. Living with someone that wasn't her husband made it worse. She came to the well at a time that no one else did. Most preachers will say this is due to her being ashamed, and people may have been bickering and talking about her and her status.

Somehow Jesus felt that he had to go to Samaria at that time. No one around him understood why he had to go there. Culturally, Jewish people had nothing to do with Samarians, and men didn't have anything to do with women who were not their wives. However, Jesus had to go to that place at that time, which leads me to believe that he came to see about her. After conversations about where she was, who she was, and her religious beliefs, I believe he changed the trajectory of her life. She dropped what she was doing and went and told everybody about Jesus. She essentially became an evangelist after meeting with Jesus. No longer ashamed; we don't even know if she went back to that man she was living with, but she began to fulfill her purpose. I believe healing took place through her talking to Jesus (therapy). I believe he built her self-esteem and changed her mindset. The well was a place of healing and transformation. That is the impact I want to bring to my community.

As a branding consultant, he heard my heart and my passion, coupled with my testimony, and said, "It sounds like you want people to meet you at the well." I thought that was quite the concept. I immediately saw the couch and myself, along with other professionals meeting people in a setting that was comfortable, inviting, and cozy to heal and set free. This tied together everything that I believed and stood for, my purpose, and my passion.

My song was inspired from my abuse but also the abuse of those girls at the hand of that famous music artist. That artist was a victim of abuse himself. If somebody would have reached him or if he received therapy after his abuse he may not have abused others. He also was a musical genius. Geniuses and the gifted fight most in their minds, like my husband, who was very talented prophetically. He was also brilliant, but there was a mental battle happening before the addictions. There was a battle all the time, and we talked about his highs and lows, him trying to see if he was enough, if he was doing the right thing, people betraying him and his traumatic childhood. He began to boast in his prophetic gift. But some of us also discovered when he would be told stuff by people and then prophesy it as if the Lord gave him the download. I've seen this a lot in ministry also. It's not right, and it should be a crime to say God said when He didn't.

I had a psychology degree and had worked with at-risk children during my first job. I then went back to school for clinical counseling to have the proper credentials to counsel in my church, and now I was back in school for counseling. It had been over 20 years of mastering my counseling career, only to experience the effects of mental illness personally. I believe God allowed this so that I would not only have the book knowledge, but the intense experience to be able to empathize with people. It didn't end there—I now work at a day rehabilitation center, counseling adults who are mentally ill.

My clients suffer from anxiety, depression, bipolar, schizophrenia, and more. I want to teach people the difference between being mentally ill and mental health awareness. We check other major parts of our body yearly, but not our minds. Millions of Americans suffer from depression and anxiety. When depression and anxiety last longer than two months and interrupt your life, it's a mental illness.

Awareness is essential, especially in cultures that don't discuss mental health (like most cultures outside of this western culture, men, and those in leadership). Most are unaware of or ashamed to admit their mental health status. Then we are shocked to find out that a pastor who was a mental health counselor committed suicide. We are so used to covering everything in church that we cover until it hurts us. Or if you have a narcissist in leadership, who emotionally abuse those in their care. People culturally accept this abuse and suffer in silence for years because they are taught if they come against it; they are coming against God.

Narcissism is an underrated conversation, and people who are abused by narcissists are sometimes unaware that they are victims. Narcissists are cunning, manipulative, and subtle. When the narcissist is aware that you see them, they demonize you to anyone that they think you will expose them. I wrote this in a blog:

- *In a relationship with a narcissist, people will never understand the trauma endured unless they have been in it themselves. You almost seem crazy for leaving or talking about the person who presented themselves as being perfect and the best thing that ever happened to you, so much so that your friends and family believe the lie (well some of them). More so, because you were manipulated into believing the lie, you helped the manipulator convince everyone around you of the same lie.*

- *One of the most toxic relationships to be in is with a narcissist. Staying in a relationship with someone that has this mental illness may cause you to end up mentally ill. They cannot be helped because they are so puffed up and arrogant, and research has shown they almost never seek help. You may find yourself depressed, having anxiety, self-doubt, low self-esteem (if you didn't already have it going in), amongst other mental battles during and after being in a relationship with a narcissist! The subtle manipulative ways of a narcissist are not talked about much; therefore, people do not know that they are emotionally abused until it's too late. As a mental health professional, it is my duty to warn you before major damage is done and to help those to heal from the effects of such a traumatic relationship. Once you know better, you can do better. You have been warned!*

"Empath," "gaslighting", "triangulation," "new supply," I found the language and articulation by following narcissist healing pages on Instagram. This was also instrumental in my healing process. Somebody understood; someone had been through this. I'm not an alien, nor am I the horrible things he said about me. Narcs not only do this in love relationships but to parents, children, staff, etc. It's a hidden epidemic. Narcissistic abuse is one of the traumas I'd love to help others get through.

Years ago, I became a Zumba and fitness instructor. My passion was not just mental wellness but became physical wellness also. As I'm writing my vision, I also know that I cannot do anything without God being the center. Although I want to reach an audience outside of the church as well as in the church, I wanted to do it in an unchurched way, but I'll never do it without God. I am a spiritual being, and I will always have a call on my life. Therefore, this is the idea that fully packaged @ The Well.

We are triune beings which means, we are spirits wrapped in a fleshly body, moved by the mind. My passion is that we are mentally (mind), physically (body), and spiritually (spirit), well. All of these parts are intertwined. If we are mentally stressed and suffer anxiety, along with other mental disorders, it affects our physical bodies. Anger, bitterness, heartbreak, can all cause stress and anxiety. Chronic stress exposes your body to unhealthy, persistently elevated levels of stress hormones like adrenaline and cortisol. Studies also link stress to changes in the way blood clots, which increases the risk of a heart attack. If our mind is intact but what we put in it is killing our bodies, we can›t even get where our minds are telling us to go. Last but certainly not least, our spirits are essential and belong to God. Therefore, we must read and understand the manual (Bible) that God has given us to live a spirit-filled life. We must understand it not according to man›s interpretation and experience, but we must read and study for ourselves.

This vision was a thought in its infant stage in early 2019. I have given up on it several times. Especially while in and out of court for child support and going through a divorce. Therefore, even though child support went into judgment. He still refused to pay it after four sporadic payments then he stopped. Oh, and for the year that he was gone, he only called when I posted that it was their birthday because he didn't remember their birthdays even when he lived with them, buying a birthday gift each. But he's telling people he pays child support, and that I'm keeping the kids from him. Lies, of course, because he wasn't asking to see them. Not that I would let him until we can prove that he is mentally stable and won't snap and hurt them. But to say I'm not letting you see them, why lie? Oh, because he has to look like the great father, he's portrayed himself to be. It's okay because I know he's obsessed with being sick and having spiders and Lyme disease, so nobody is a priority. Nonetheless, the lies are consistent with his way to manipulate and keep the people around him sympathizing with him. Narcissist crave attention and sympathy.

So, the ups and downs of that, working, going to school, mourning my marriage, mourning my church, and the life I once knew, I didn't always want to follow through with this vision. However, connecting with people who would confirm it was my push to keep moving forward. But then I fought with the fact that I felt like I failed in my life, and no one would want to hear from someone whose marriage fell apart and couldn't even help her husband. That was still my guilt. Which I am now free of because you can't help one who doesn't want to be helped. Furthermore, you can't keep helping someone else at your own expense.

With this book, I not only want to bring education and awareness to being well, but I want people to understand that my passion comes from my experience. It's one thing to have the book knowledge and the vocational experience, but people want to hear from someone who's been through it and can walk them through coming out. When I have my workshops and my meetings, I want it to be a setting outside of the church and one of a wellness atmosphere. I want all to feel welcome and ready to share, help, and get help. I want people to be able to ask questions. We have enough women's conferences, men's conferences, youth conferences. My greatest joy was when I had a girl talks at my church, and people were able to ask questions, and I was able to be transparent with them about my life. I was always told that it helped more than someone preaching at them. Preaching is good, getting a greater understanding of the word and its application is incredible. How can they hear except they have a preacher? I do agree. However, working with people in small groups and one-on-one has always been a great joy for me and yielded more results in my ministry.

The great thing about everything that has taken place is that I know that God allowed it for my purpose. People who knew what was going on wondered how I came through all of that with my mind intact. I often say, I lost it and got it back; or some days it's not all there, trust me. And I almost died in it. As I was going through my healing process, my education in my vocation kept me in the state of a mental health check. Sometimes I would wake up and be shaken in the middle of the night from the trauma that I have survived. Sometimes I would not be able to sleep. As I was counseling my clients and giving them the tools such as guided meditations for positive affirmation and positive energy and meditations for better sleep, I realized I was giving them tools that I could use for myself as well, and I did. Everything I was reading in my courses I made sure to use in my own life. One of the first things we learn in counseling is that we must see a therapist also and to constantly check our mental state in the process of counseling others. God orchestrated my vocation and my education to make sure that I was well.

My heart was broken in the situation, but the healing process was fantastic. Someone asked me if I would get married again. Directly after the ordeal I experienced, my answer was no, but now, two years later, my answer is absolutely. I think that having a companion is wonderful, but this time around, I know who I am, I know what I want and what I don't want. I believe in our twenties; we think we know what we want, but we haven't been around on this earth long enough, nor around enough people to even be able to make that decision.

I'm grateful for the future. I'm thankful for the people that hung out with me while I was in the trenches. Although I'm not mentioning names in this book, they know who they are. After the attack and the public embarrassment, there were a handful who stayed close in the most critical season of my life. My best friend who has always been there and would check up on me at least weekly or so to make sure I was good and tell me I was going to be alright and that all would be well. She always knew how to make me laugh and feel better about my life, no matter where I was. Money, court, long talks, she's the sister I never knew I needed.

Then there's a young lady who would help with all the systems and events that I put together in the church. She was like my secretary. She was pulling her life together and had just graduated with her clinical counseling degree when this all went down. Again, I couldn't afford therapy, but the people, places, and things He placed around me were priceless. She understood clinically what I went through and what I had experienced. We walked and talked through all of my trauma. She called weekly to make sure I was good after my attack, and she brought her kids around so they would have each other and her profession and mine collided, so she is a member on the board of @ The Well.

I'm thankful for one of the brothers with whom I was accused of having an affair. This thing rocked us both because our names were being blasted on Facebook and YouTube and almost drove us crazy. People were calling us and asking us questions. It was especially life-changing. He also retreated but made sure to check in on me weekly, sometimes daily. We talked to each other through the insanity it almost caused us. It was also great talking to someone who saw the before and after, someone who believed in his ministry at one time but had also seen the manipulation and abuse. He was also part of the handful that knew I tried to commit suicide and didn't want to see me go that route again. Not only was he willing to talk about fighting on my behalf, but he was ready to physically fight on my behalf, along with the prayer and the ministry on his life that got me through some of the hard days. I'm forever grateful that he remains a confidant and friend to this day.

Then my big sister/girlfriend, who is an evangelist and started as my husband's best friend. I could just call her crying, and she would ask no questions, but just start praying. She helped me to rationalize through my thoughts. I love talking to her because she knew him before me and experienced all that I saw going on behind the scenes firsthand. Her brother, and I all suffered from PTSD after these events. Also, the doubts fears, and his negatives words are something we fight collectively and individually to this day. We realized outside of him; we will make it; we aren't weak, dumb, and incompetent. We also mourned the potential we saw in him. We mourned the church that we helped to build with our blood, sweat, and tears. She got it. I didn't always have to express or explain what I experienced, felt, or the pain I did. She would just come and get my kids, and like the others, sensed when I was in need, emotionally, financially, and spiritually. She would come to the house and just chill. As a life coach, she walked me through my vision, goals, and planned to see it to manifestation.

My family, as always, was there. We didn't have to see each other every day, but when I called, they were right there, my mom, my dad, my aunt, cousins, sister, and brother. And let's not talk about all my uncles to whom I still give limited information because I don't want them to have to hurt anybody. They never allow me to walk into a courtroom alone. Even though he was a no-show most times, prolonging every case, I had anxiety every time I thought I would see him. There were a few more people that were there that started to dwindle away to get back into their own life but checked in here and there, like those ladies who saw the trauma up close and actually were victims to the trauma. We all needed therapy after what we witnessed. There were some ministers from our church and others who checked in now and then also. Some members and folks from other churches continued to invite me places to make sure I was good.

Of course, I heard others were talking about me. But I could care less. I was grateful that God revealed who was for me and who was not in this season. Some kept their distance. When I was on a platform going up and high in ministry, I had people that just wanted to walk with me while I was going up. But when the limelight stopped shining, I had strangers supporting me more than the people who claimed to love me and to be riding for me. What I am clear of is some people are in our lives for seasons, and then their time is up. This is perfectly okay. It's not always malicious, either. There were people that I was close to, and then I had to move to where God was calling me to next. I am not upset with anyone. I'm sometimes still disappointed in my husband's actions. I realize it wasn't personal, as anyone in his way could get this treatment, from his momma down to his children. It is a sickness.

When I decided to go back out to concerts and church services, some of my colleagues and those with whom I fellowshipped, sang and preached for would be so happy to see me and see that I was okay. They would tell me how they didn't want to call because they were afraid of appearing nosy, so they prayed from afar. That helped me. I wondered why I knew so many bishops, pastors, and pastors' wives, and only a handful called me before I changed my number. Even after changing my number, people would inbox me prayers when they couldn't reach me. But I do understand how if you didn't call me before this, then calling me after would be awkward.

Last but certainly not least, I owe my young branding consultant for helping me to rebuild and rebrand myself. For all the advertisements, his belief in my vision, and for not charging nearly what it cost to do the work he did for me when I didn't have the funds to get started. It's one thing for people to do work for you and not be attached to the vision, but to have someone see and visualize where I was going, and capture it visually was a blessing. Not to mention him having an ear when business conversations turned into me venting about my complicated life. I can now also call him a friend.

Now, after I decided to start putting up my social media content, the calls started coming in. I was asked to speak at a few events. I didn't have all the money I needed, but my CPA allowed a payment plan to incorporate my non-for-profit, @ The Well Wellness Center Inc. I knew I wanted to move in excellence, but I didn't have all the finances that I needed to get it going. But as I begin to tell people what I was doing, they offered to be donators and sponsors. Everyone I spoke to agreed that this conversation and the services are needed. Some people offered and donated their time, services, and expertise. I was going to launch earlier, but finances and cold feet made me push the date back several times. However, once I committed, everything divinely started to come together.

I am here now. With some help from that young branding consultant, I got on all of my social media sites. I rebuilt the face of Lady J. I was going to pay someone to build my website, but I almost forgot that when I take my time to learn programs, I can be so determined that I'll stay up all night to learn every aspect of it. So, I built my website. I changed my name because I felt like he embarrassed our name. Every time you typed in my married name, that horrible live event on Facebook came up. I didn't want to be known for that, so I went back to my maiden name. That is why I have no problem with sharing and being transparent, even for those who know me reading this book. Mostly everything that I disclosed he had already exposed live on Facebook, and over the pulpit.

My freedom is here, my new beginning is now. I am now an author, the CEO and founder of a nonprofit, working on my master›s degree with my doctorate to follow and still raising my beautiful children with the help of family and friends. There›s a whole new world ahead of me. If I could make it through all that I made it through, rebuild and rebrand myself after such a horrific trial in my life, there's nothing I can't do if I put my mind to it. I felt that before at times, but I know it for sure now.

I've always been resilient, and I can't stop now.

I could not shield my children from this trauma. I tried for as long as I could until it was apparent that something was not right. However, what I will show them is that after all that their mommy endured, she is still successful. Moreover, these trials made her the strong, powerful, and successful woman she is today. It's not so much what you've been through that shapes you, (because it could shape you negatively and positively) but it's what you learn and make of it that makes you phenomenal. I could have hidden away and became a basket case or lived a mediocre life, which is where I wanted to settle so many times. But I chose to use my trials for the purpose placed on me before the foundation of the world. It only added to my resume.

As for suicide, it's almost always a big shock to everyone that a person committed suicide. People are like, "Wait a minute, not them!" Often, people who carry out suicide are those that most of the time, they don't tell you they're going to do it. It's those who are seeking attention or crying out for help who make an announcement. I have a client with Borderline Personality Disorder who has suicidal ideations. She tells every staff member that she wants to kill herself until she gets the attention she wants. She learned what to say to force us to call the hospital immediately. The hospital is the ultimate attention, but she has never actually attempted.

However, those who follow through often keep their thoughts to themselves over time, and when the opportunity presents itself with some reinforcements such as stress, trauma, abuse, and drug abuse, and with one thought, they are gone. These people don't believe they have a safe place to talk about their issues as culture has told them it is weak to have these feelings (like in church or the African American community). In other cases, the weight of a family or company is too much. People are expecting them to be strong, and they can't afford to be weak. All of the above applied to me.

This is why I want to open the conversation on mental health and suicide. We have to normalize this because so many suffer in silence. If we normalize these topics, people will not be afraid to cry out for help. One of my first Facebook live videos was about suicide, and the response was great.

I hope that this book can reach others—even if it is just one. If one person doubting will change their mind or if it stops one person from committing suicide, or if it helps one relationship, I will be happy. If it helps one woman decide not to take abuse, or if it helps a woman in her relationship or marriage see the signs of her significant other suffering with depression/anxiety before it gets too late, I will be happy.

Finally, I want everyone reading this book to know that no matter what you're going through, keep moving forward so you can come out. Know and believe that you can make it through anything. I will never forget what I went through; therefore, I recognize that I am susceptible to mental battles. However, I'm willing and able to fight back. I have the tools I need now to get through it. I have a support system, my children, my story, and I know that helping others is going to be a part of the continual healing and what frees me and makes me whole. I was at my best when I was helping other people, doing what God called me to do. I took some time off and had some time away from people because I needed that. I needed to discover who I was again. I needed to hear my voice again. I needed to hear God's voice for myself again. I needed that space and time, that quiet, isolated space to develop into the woman that I had been becoming, who I am, and who I am constantly evolving. I wholeheartedly believe that the next phase of my life will be extraordinary. I'll have a remarkable story of what has come of all of this. The next 40 will be my best 40!

CPSIA information can be obtained
at www.ICGtesting.com
Printed in the USA
FSHW011941200320
68286FS

9 781648 260711